Christ
Centered
Childbirth

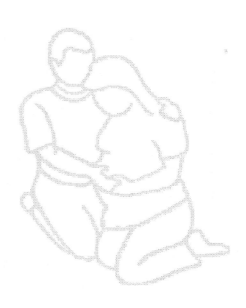

Kelly J. Townsend

Christ Centered Childbirth

Kelly J. Townsend

Forward
Petar-Krešimir Hodžić, M.D.

Four Winds Publications
PO Box 3004
Gilbert, AZ 85299

Christ Centered Childbirth
© 2001, 2005 Kelly J. Townsend   All rights reserved.

This book is a work of non-fiction. Unless otherwise noted, the author and the publisher make no explicit guarantees as to the accuracy of the information contained in this book and in some cases, names of people and places have been changed to protect their privacy. No information contained in this book is meant to diagnose or treat any medical condition and is not to be construed as such. The author accepts no liability of the medical outcome of any pregnancy or birth, and this book is intended as a guide for spiritual edification alone.

No part of this book may be reproduced, stored in a retrieval system, or transmitted by any means without the written permission from the author.

First published by Four Winds Publications 07/31/05

ISBN: 978-0-9769505-0-9

Printed in the United States of America

Scripture taken from the
HOLY BIBLE, NEW INTERNATIONAL VERSION
Copyright © 1973, 1978, 1984 by International Bible Society
Used by permission of Zondervan Publishing House, All rights reserved.

The "NIV" and "New International Version" trademarks are registered in the United States Patent and Trademark Office by the International Bible Society. Use of either trademark requires the permission of International Bible Society."

All clipart copyright © Microsoft Word 2002
Cover photo copyright © Ellen Bauman 2003
This book is printed on acid-free paper

This book is dedicated to Jesus Christ, my first true love, my dear husband Dan, and my sweet children.

I would also like to dedicate this book to
the late Dr. Grantly Dick-Read,
the pioneer of modern natural childbirth.
May his work continue to bless us,
and may he never be forgotten…

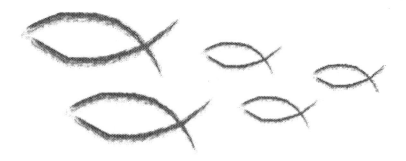

All the ends of the earth
will remember and turn to the LORD,

and all the families of the nations
will bow down before him,

for dominion belongs to the LORD
and he rules over the nations.

Psalm 22:27-28

Table of Contents

www.ChristCenteredChildbirth.com

Acknowledgments

First, and foremost, I would like to thank Jesus Christ for the grace He has given me, for His sacrifice, and for His will to allow this book to happen. I am forever thankful to Him!

Secondly, I want to thank my dear husband, Dan Townsend, for his patience with me, his sacrifice, and his love during this five-year project. You must really love me! I also want to thank my children for being patient too, we have been through the heavy trenches, but had a lot of fun mud wars while we were there! You guys always know how to have fun!

I could not have written this book without all the loving advice from all of my colleagues, helping me edit and refine this work in progress. I especially want to mention Penny Juaregui, my good friend and mentor. How could I have navigated this without you? Shawna McKinnis also was very instrumental in the foundational work when this all began. Her friendship is above rubies to me. In addition, I wanted to thank all the pastors at Applegate Christian Fellowship for putting up with my many phone calls asking about doctrine. You guys are awesome!

I would like to mention all the readers over the years whose testimonies have encouraged me to continue on. Of particular importance to me are the readers Petar-Krešimir Hodžić M.D., and his wife Rafaela, who have touched my ministry in such a profound way that I could never express. Their tireless work with the families of Croatia has been such an inspiration and a blessing to me. They have been faithfully spreading the news about the Croatian version of Christ Centered Childbirth throughout their country, and the Lord continues to bless many women over there, thanks to them.

Finally, I would like to thank my very good friend Jennifer Vanderlaan for her honesty and professionalism, which prodded and inspired me to go that extra step. The hours spent on the phone are priceless to me, and I look forward to many more years of growth as colleagues and friends. Thanks, Jen!

Preface

Father God, we come before you and ask that you would be the Lord of our family, and we follow Your truths and Your ways. We ask You for a blessing, and please be with us as we seek to be fruitful. Help us to prepare, to be responsible, and not to fear – we know You have given us this baby, and You will help us provide for him. Go before us and prepare the way, and we ask this in Jesus' name, Amen!

What a wonderful God we serve! He is so gracious to give us the ability to be the vessel used to bring forth such a fantastic work of art called life. Yet, what do we really do to cause this little child to come into being? We have found out how to place a child in the womb, but can we knit him together? No, life still belongs in the hand of the Creator. It is a marvelous thing to consider; that awesome work of our Father still deserves our praise. Let us sing hallelujah and go to our knees in adoration of such a great King who is awesome in power, yet personal and loving, giving us the privilege to carry His artwork. He even gives us a small role to play in the process, and this book is designed to help us navigate the waters of creation, going responsibly forward toward our goal of a larger family. Children are a blessing, perhaps more than we will ever know...

My prayers are with you, and I pray you will find what you are looking for here. I encourage you to be diligent in your search for knowledge and edification, discerning and wise as you sift through the mountains of literature and media. Keep in mind always that God sustained His people long before there was a printing press or a television to watch a movie about birth or parenting. He has placed within you the instinct needed to rear children, but has also given you a free will to make the choices. Go forth carefully with reverence for the Lord, choosing His excellent ways, and you will not be disappointed.

As for me, far be it from me that I should sin against the LORD by failing to pray for you. And I will teach you the way that is good and right. [24] But be sure to fear the LORD and serve him faithfully with all your heart; consider what great things he has done for you.

1Samuel 12:23-24

Note From The Author

I am the Alpha and the Omega, the First and the Last,
the Beginning and the End. Revelation 22:13

On the book cover, you will see the symbols of the Alpha and the Omega, the first and last letter of the Greek alphabet, surrounding the laboring couple as she peacefully breathes through a contraction. Jesus told us that He is the beginning of all that we are allowed to do, and that He will be there to the very end, never leaving our side. May this book be an encouragement to you to place Jesus Christ at the beginning of your pregnancy, and may He be a dominating figure in your family's life until the end of your parenting career. May every decision and action you take begin with prayer and petition to Him, and may you rest in the knowledge that He goes before you in all situations, and is also behind you as your Protector. Above all else, may your pregnancy, labor and delivery be filled with the resurrection power that will erupt in pure joy as you gaze into the eyes of your new family member for the first time.

The Purpose Of This Book

This book is primarily designed to bring you closer to Jesus Christ. It is not so much a medical manual to help you through the physical aspects of birth (although there is basic and very useful information about the process), but it is meant to be a spiritual guide for you, the Christian couple, as you enter the most excellent career of your life, parenthood. Use this book as a study guide, an edification tool, and a Bible study tool. You may choose to use each chapter as a Bible study topic, with discussion topics at the end of each chapter. Read it at least twice, and enjoy the blessings of participating in a beautiful miracle of God. Be blessed, and happy birthing!

Forward

Dr. Petar-Krešimir Hodžić
Zagreb, Croatia

What is truth? Where is light? Many of us will shout those questions in an attempt to find a solid anchor in our lives. Without a doubt, we are living in a world where basic human values are being constantly undermined by a technocratic lifestyle infused with consumerism. At the same time, the hectic rhythm of our daily obligations is depriving us of those precious moments when we can look into the depths of our being, searching for true meaning and purpose.

Are we ready to start asking ourselves about the meaning of procreation and childbirth as potentially life transforming events in a woman's life? In today's technological climate of childbirth, many have found that those life-transforming moments can sometimes be buried below the layers of accumulated fears, misconceptions, and prejudices. What they hoped for was a rich well of blessing that every women dreams of about birth. Instead, the spirituality of childbirth has been slowly forgotten, as faith has been set aside and hopes have been placed into the hands of man instead of God. Each woman does have within herself the ability to tap in to that well of supernatural strength needed to accomplish the birth with peace and joy, if given the opportunity.

Women all over the world need a caring hand and nurturing support during processes of childbirth. The question is if there is anyone out there to give them that hand, and if the human hand is enough. We are witnessing various epidemics of fear, but the epidemic of fear during childbirth is spreading over the world like a plague that calls for immediate action. Healthcare professionals, especially in Scandinavia, are doing extensive research on the medical and psychological aspects related to fear of childbirth, and the importance of reducing the phobia of birth, yet still they have found no definitive and simple solution to the complex problem.

The complexity and beauty of the natural childbirth process is so vividly evident when the hormonal orchestration is examined. The beautiful balance of the biological symphony is made of cocktail of hormones and body chemicals like estrogen, progesterone, oxytocin, prolactin, beta-endorphins and cateholamines. Among them, oxytocin (the hormone of love) and prolactin (the hormone of mothering), may play the most critical role setting the foundation of confident and nurturing motherhood.

During the normal and undisturbed action of giving birth, these hormones are circulating in a balanced proportion that is just right for that particular mother. This type of labor and delivery, where basic conditions of security and privacy are fulfilled, is now an unreachable ideal for millions of women worldwide. The fear of a painful labor, creating a certain cycle of self-fulfilling prophecy, is spinning fast in many ladies and due to the multiple disturbances during labor, including many routine interventions, women are being deprived of the normal hormonal effects on their brain that occur otherwise.

What does it mean, then, for women when those hormonal seals of love and mothering are cut out from their childbirth experience? We may only wonder what the spiritual consequences might be, and how that might affect the level of human existence that could be possible if we were to allow the normal process of labor and delivery to take its course.

With this in mind, my wife and I began searching the available literature in order to find as many books, tips and ideas that would help us in preparation for the birth of our own child. Although we had read many excellent books on that subject, something was continuously missing. When I found Kelly Townsend's e-book, Christ Centered Childbirth, we knew that our search had ended. The book profoundly touched the core of our being and our belief system. As Christians, we immediately decided to translate it and to make it available to all women in Croatia. Since the book has been published in 2003 we have received numerous testimonies from women regarding how the book changed their perspective and helped them retain the joy and beauty of childbirth despite the circumstances. Therefore, we now have valuable testimonies and stories for the second edition of the book, including the unforgettable birth of our daughter.

Herewith, I would like to emphasize the importance of husband support during childbirth, but also the importance of the attendance of the doula. The serious studies confirmed that need, in terms of birth course and birth outcome. We are looking forward to the organization of a formal doula training project in Croatia, as we currently do not have that profile of birth professional in Croatia at all.

One might ask what is so special about the book you are holding in your hands. There is someone very special engraved into pages of the book, His name is Jesus Christ and He is the central figure. The author invites women and those supporting them to put Him in the center of their birth, and to trust Him that they are safe in His hands. In exchange,

He will preserve the joyful experience of childbirth that will transform lives to be more like Him each day.

By receiving His abundant love, we will be able to love more and the children of tomorrow will carry that love to make a better world. In this context, Kelly Townsend's book is a prophetic but practical contribution to that better world. I am sure every woman and their husband, by reading it together, could benefit from it, if only they are willing to go deeper into text. To achieve that, this book should be read at least twice by both parents, and ought to become an integral part of the inventory that pregnant women and their husbands will take to the labor site.

Let Us Pray…

Father, You are awesome beyond any words that we could ever record. May Your Holy Spirit come now into the heart of this reader to teach and to counsel, so that Your will would be done. Bless this time of reading and learning, give them a heart that is receptive to Your word, as well as discernment to recognize Your truth. Lord, calm their mind with your Holy Spirit and allow them to go confidently in the knowledge of Your redemption and grace. Cast out all fear from their minds and place a hedge of protection around them so that they might be encouraged and confident in You. Above all Lord, may you be glorified in Your people, and may this birth be a testimony of Your love and faithfulness. You are our living God, and we invite you now into this time of worship as we learn of Your ways as they relate to childbirth. Your little children declare Your love, so establish Your love in the life of this child. We praise You and thank you in the name of Your Son, Jesus Christ. Amen!

Chapter One
Love Begins at Conception

The journey of pregnancy is possibly the most sacred gift God has given to us. It is overwhelming to ponder how the Lord would consider us, when granting temporary custody of His children. Yet because of His loving kindness, a growing soul is within us and we take pleasure to do all that we can to build this very special little person. We understand that our body is the temple of the Lord, but even more amazing is the fact that we have been granted permission to take part in constructing a new little temple inside of us for Him.

We have the opportunity to pray for our baby even before conception, because the Lord knows their name and hears our prayers. Bathed in prayer, of course, is the best beginning we could possibly give. We can bring all kinds of petitions and requests to Him regarding the baby, as well as pray for all those who will touch their life, such as a future spouse, grandchildren, etc.

As our prayers unfold for our new family member, so too does our early love for her. Amazingly, studies have now shown that even the thoughts the mother has toward the baby largely affect their mental well-being in the future.[1] Her blood-borne emotional chemicals cross the placenta and the baby feels what she is feeling. Love or resentment is detected by the baby, shaping their little souls from early on. Knowing that they are loved and accepted is an important step towards positively training up our children in the ways of the Lord.

As pregnancy progresses, our attention begins to focus on the delivery. It is important to compare the possibilities for the upcoming birth with that of being born again. Every person's walk with the Lord is different, and some are born again quickly and easily, while others seem to struggle over time. No one knows for sure who will surrender to Jesus right away or who will need more time, but God knows. Much the same, each birth is different from any other, and we won't know what will happen for our birth until that blessed day.

There is a rainbow of possibilities for labor and delivery, and each color is extremely beautiful. The most important aspect of birth is that the Father is glorified and that Jesus Christ is at the center, no matter what happens. Of course, we strive to have the most complication-free delivery, with as little intervention as possible. We responsibly do that by educating ourselves of the *true* pro's and con's of each procedure, and move forward out of love for the baby in the decisions that we make. Once we do that, we place our faith in Jesus Christ that He alone is the author of our birth, and we place our trust fully in Him.

As you study all that you can about the birth of your child, make sure to be faithful in studying the Word of God. There is something special about taking in scripture through your eyes, soaking it in yourself as you study directly from the Bible. It is a very healthy thing to do when you dedicate five minutes a day to the reading of scripture, and I cannot emphasize enough how enriching it is to your walk with the Lord. The Bible likens the scriptures to water that washes you,[2] and truly reading the words written in the Bible with you own eyes almost feels fluid, as if you were drinking in living water that refreshes your soul. Let me encourage you to include the reading of scripture every day, exercising your devotional muscles.

"...and every...house divided against itself shall not stand." Matt 12:25

Husbands, may I encourage you to do all that you can to ensure unity in your marriage? As leader of your household, you have the privilege of being the covering to your wife, to be her strong tower and sanctuary during this time of your developing family. She is not the only one becoming a parent, and you are remembered and given high honor in your role regarding the growth of this baby within the womb. The best thing that you can contribute to is your dedication to strengthening the marriage. Parenthood is the noblest career ever given, and it thrives with the participation and support of a loving and understanding spiritual leader.

Make Jesus your number one priority, and study how He loved those in the church. Remember, He died for them. This might be a season of dying to yourself and your own needs, out of the love for your wife. Not to a point of extreme deprivation, however, because you are also loved by the Lord and have specific needs, as you become a new parent.

Remember to wash you wife daily in the water of the Word, covering her in prayer, and protect her from all things negative.[2] Your high calling as the pastor of your growing home is exciting and extremely rewarding beyond measure.

Parents Prior to Conception

*My frame was not hidden from you when I was made in the secret place.
When I was woven together in the depths of the earth, your eyes saw my
unformed body. All the days ordained for me were written in your book
before one of them came to be.*
Psalm 139:15-16

It would seem that our marvelous Lord wanted to father us long before we were ever conceived. He makes sure that we know we were chosen by Him to be loved and cherished until we returned home forever. Out of His love, He has afforded us the same opportunity with our own children. No doubt, you have already begun the parenting process to raise this child. The mere fact that you are already preparing for childbirth is a loving act of early parenting.

In all things, we want to model ourselves after our Lord, Jesus Christ. What a fantastic concept it is that we can now pray for this little child, for their salvation, for their health, for their peace, and for their provision. The Christian is able to step into a pre-defined role of the parent, demonstrated to us by God Himself, and begin to form a relationship with them, perhaps even before they are conceived. It is more important than ever to have a deep and personal bond with our children, and God is showing us that it starts even before conception.

It is never too late to begin the bonding process. Start right now and begin the fascinating journey of becoming the protector and intercessor for your child. Every time you send a prayer for your child, you add another stone to the tower of love that is strong beyond imagination, and is essential for her total health. Nutrition, exercise, and lifestyle are great pillars you will be constructing, but forming a love relationship with your child through prayer, communication, and touch are the building materials that will ensure a lifetime of joy.

*Before I formed you in the womb I knew you,
before you were born I set you apart...*
Jeremiah 1:5

Father God, we know that You are eternal, and that You are in the past right now, as well as the future. Please place Your hand of protection over all that has been done in the process of forming this child. Just the same, You are right now looking at what has already

23

been established and we ask that You would give a special blessing to this child. Lord, truly You can move throughout the framework of time and so go into the future and place a hedge of protection around this precious child. Help us, as parents, to grow daily in deeper love with them. May every decision that we make be for their benefit. May we become the parents that You called us to be, and may You show us moment by moment that the most excellent way of parenting is with love.

Prenatal Communication

As we deepen our love for the baby, our decisions shift from seeking the solution that best suits our own needs, to that which will best benefit the baby. A season of "setting the self aside" gets off to a good start when we become acquainted early on with our newest family member through prenatal communication. This can happen through many activities, including prayer, stories, singing a familiar set of songs, external fetal massage, and fetal rocking.

Activities To Try

Top of the hour talk – Make it a habit, starting from conception, to spend 3-5 minutes at the top of each hour to communicate something to your baby. Tell her about your love, whether it is in voice or in spirit, as you would if you were holding her in your arms.

Rocking Music – Pick a favorite song or lullaby, and sing it to baby while you gently rock him with your hips. Use the same songs that you plan on rocking him to sleep with once he has been born. Babies enjoy familiarity, and it is never too soon to start.

Play-Time Music – Develop your own play games with the baby that you will perform to music. Choose children's Sunday school songs and combine them with specific hand motions on the abdomen. Marry the hand movements with the song, so that each time you have a performance, the baby will be able to anticipate the action, giving him a sense of predictability and routine. Once baby is born, perform the same movements in person.

Jesus Loves Me (Chorus Only)

"Jesus loves me, this I know,
(Rub the sides of your belly from the back to the front in rhythm)

For the Bible tells me so.
(Hug your belly and gently rock side to side)

Little ones to Him belong,
(Repeat step one)

They are weak but He is strong."
(Repeat step two)

The B-I-B-L-E

"The B-I-B-L-E,
(Pat the left side of your belly in rhythm of the song)

Yes that's the book for me,
(Pat the lower middle of your belly in rhythm of the song)

I stand upon the Word of God,
(Pat the Right side of your belly in rhythm of the song)

The B-I-B-L-E,
(Pat the top of your belly in rhythm of the song)

Bible!"
(Hug your belly & gently rock it as you exclaim "Bible!)

He's Got the Whole World In His Hands

He's got the whole world in his hands
(Rub a big circle around your stomach)

He's got the itty bitty babies in his hands
(Cradle belly and rock baby)

He's got the mommies and the daddies in his hands

(Mom sings "mommies" and pats belly on left and Dad sings "daddies" and pats belly on right)

He's got the whole world in his hands
(Repeat step one, both parents singing)

This Little Light of Mine
(Use a flashlight near baby's head and place on different areas throughout the song)

This little light of mine, I'm gonna let it shine

This little light of mine, I'm gonna let it shine

This little light of mine, I'm gonna let it shine

Let it shine, let it shine, let it shine.

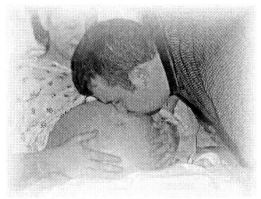

Photo Courtesy of Crystal Skidmore

Worship

Just as emotions can cross the placental barrier, so too can spiritual worship. There is power in heart-felt worship, with a mind focused on the immediate presence of the Lord. This can manifest itself in many ways, including joining others in the singing of worship music, lifting hands, and outward expressions or inward meditations of love and praise of the Lord.

26

Identify Your Baby

Although it has become fashionable and convenient to find out the gender of the baby before birth through ultrasound, many parents are returning to the design of the Father in waiting for the birth to know the sex of the baby. For those parents, it can be a good idea to create some kind of nickname for either a male of female. For example, one baby's parents called him "Baby J" during the pregnancy. They planned on giving him his father's name if it was a boy, making him a Junior, and if it were to be a girl, naming her Joy. The extended family was then able to bond with the idea of "Baby J," even addressing cards to him with that name, making it easier to wait until birth to find out.

Have fun incorporating these games into your daily routine with baby. Set your inhibitions aside and really get to know this child early. You will be so glad you did. May we, as parents, pour out our love and not hold back. Abundant love and faith for our Father surrounds us. Let us work to form a life-long bond which begins in the womb!

I would like to extend special thanks to Dr. Petar-Krešimir and Rafaela Hodžić of Croatia for demonstrating these ideas and principles with enormous and complete love to their unborn baby. Their love of God, of each other, and their daughter made an obvious difference in their birth experience, and was visible in their postpartum interactions. They considered themselves not parents-to-be, but rather parents from conception, and perhaps before. What I witnessed there has forever affected my belief that prenatal bonding is paramount.

1. Maternal Emotions and Human Development By Bruce H. Lipton, Ph.D. (1995)
2. Ephesians 5:26

Bible Study Discussion

1. How have you bonded with your baby so far?

2. Perform some of the songs in this chapter for your baby.

3. Have you given your baby a nick-name yet?

4. What are you doing to show your baby that you love them?

5. How are you controlling stress?

Chapter Two
The Author of Life

Asking For A Family

How many stories have you heard of women who tried to get pregnant for years, finally adopted, and then conceived? I, myself, tried for 11 months to conceive and after finally giving up, and then on the twelfth month conceived my oldest daughter.

I do not want to be the one to tell you exactly how you should go about conception, but I would like to encourage you to seek the Lord and see what His will would be in your life. Take a very close look at the difference between His perfect will, and His permissive will. God allows things in our lives that might not have been His perfect plan, and it might not be what is best for us. Let us always strive to achieve His perfect will, so that our joy might be full.

Remember, God is eternal. Eternity is not only now and forever, but also His ability to be outside the framework of time, and able to look upon the events in the past, the present, and the future simultaneously. Why not, then, ask Him to heal those things in your past that He can see right now, and then ask Him to bless you and your family as He looks upon them in the future this very moment?

Natural Conception

There are many ways the Lord has given us to assess our fertility, and we can take notice of those indications in order to increase the possibility of pregnancy. The following are some very basic indicators of fertility:

- Cervical Mucous – If you haven't already, start paying attention to the nature of your cervical mucous (discharge) throughout your menstrual cycle. In order for the seed to travel to the egg, the mucous needs to be thin enough for easy swimming! You will notice around the middle of your cycle (assuming your cycles are normal) that your cervical mucous becomes more of a liquid. This is a good sign that you are fertile.
- Saliva/cervical mucous testing – A little secret that is becoming more well known. You can purchase a personal ovulation

microscope, which analyzes your saliva upon drying. When a woman is about to ovulate, there will be a ferning pattern to her dried saliva and/or cervical mucous that can be seen under a simple microscope. Fertility-Focus is a company that makes a small microscope that looks like a tube of lipstick that you can keep in your purse and track your fertility daily. The cost is about 25.00-30.00 dollars.

- Libido – It isn't surprising to note that a woman might have an increase in libido before she ovulates. Pay attention to your libido in combination with these other indications to see if there is a change.

- Basal Body Temperature – If your cycles are normal, then you might be able to use this method to predict ovulation. Track your basal body temperature, the temperature you have in the morning prior to becoming active, with a basal thermometer. You will notice a slight increase in temperature, then a sudden drop followed by an increase in temperature that should last the rest of your cycle. It is when the sudden drop happens that you should be fertile.

- Urine Test – You can purchase ovulation predictor tests that test your urine for a hormone that signals fertility. These can be quite pricey; however, I have seen them in abundance at the dollar store!

The Struggles

We have an abundance of estrogen in our world, from the dairy, eggs, and meat we eat that is loaded with it for production reasons, to the soy products, and even in the water we drink tainted by estrogen coming from birth control pills that does not get filtered at the water plant. One of the problems is Polycystic Ovarian Disease (PCOS), which causes multiple eggs to develop but rarely any actually get released to the fallopian tube, is too much estrogen and not enough progesterone. I highly recommend reading "What Your Doctor May Not Tell You About Pre-menopause" by Dr. John Lee. In this book, he explains the problem with the deficiency of natural progesterone and it's role in polycystic ovarian disease and infertility.

Women who are having difficulty conceiving may want to look at the symptoms of PCOS if they have not considered this as a possibility.

- Infrequent menstrual periods, irregular periods, or irregular bleeding
- Infertility
- Increased growth of hair on the face, chest, stomach, back, thumbs or toes
- Acne, oily skin, Skin tags, or dandruff
- Pelvic pain
- Weight gain or obesity, carrying the weight around the waist
- Type 2 diabetes
- High Cholesterol
- High Blood Pressure
- Thin hair
- Patches of dark skin on the neck, arms, breasts, or thighs
- Sleep apnea – Snoring with the cessation of breathing at times during sleep

This is not meant to diagnose, but is placed here to give those with the above symptoms an opportunity to discuss the issue with their health care provider. Take a good look at your diet, your life style, and your reproductive health to make sure that your body is completely prepared for pregnancy. God has the perfect time for you to become pregnant. In the meantime, make sure you are parenting your child by preparing your womb to be the healthiest place possible.

When You Cannot Become Pregnant

The Bible does not come right out and tell us what to do in this situation, except to pray for God to have favor upon us in blessing us with a child. You can take the problem into your own hands, and look to man to provide a child by artificial means. This is something you are going to have to reconcile with God, because the Bible does say that He is the Author of life in the book of Acts, and it is important to really pray over what that means.

Let's look at a well-known couple who took matters into their own hands. In the book of Genesis, faithful Abraham heard God's promise that his seed would outnumber the stars in the sky. He became impatient, however, and wondered if he needed to help God, so-to-speak, by having relations with His maid-servant and Ishmael was born. Sara did conceive, at an old age, and Isaac was the promised child. The twelve tribes of Israel were born from Isaac, through Jacob, and of course, then, the lineage to Jesus Christ. What happened to Ishmael? His descendants have been traced to a religion that claims that Ishmael was the chosen son, and that religion has been at battle with the Jews ever since.

My point? Be careful taking things into your own hands by "helping out God." I am not saying that any intervention is going to cause an Ishmael in your life, but be very careful that you remain within God's perfect will, not His permissive will.

In all things, make your family building enjoyable! There is loveliness to creation, and being caught up in the science of it all can really make it a chore rather than a joy. Relax, and have fun!

Quiet Moment:

Consider all of the great things the Lord has done for you so far. How has He taken care of you in the difficult times in your life? Tell the Lord that you will put your faith in the fact that He will provide you with what you need, at exactly the time you need it. Tell Him you trust Him, and that all you want is what He wants for you, and that you pass the reins of your life over to Him, giving Him all control....

He Has Found Favor – You're Pregnant!

Mary's Song

"And Mary said; 'My soul glorifies the Lord and my spirit rejoices in God my Savior, for he has been mindful of the humble state of his servant. From now on all generations will call me blessed, for the Mighty One has done great things for me- holy is his name. His mercy extends to those who fear him, from generation to generation. He has performed mighty deeds with his arm; he has scattered those who are proud in their innermost thoughts. He has brought down rulers from their thrones but has lifted up the humble. He has filled the hungry with good things but has sent the rich away empty. He has helped his servant Israel, remembering to be merciful to Abraham and his descendants forever, even as he said to our fathers.' Luke 1:46-55

How we love you, Lord! Thank you so much for your provision, You have provided this child! We ask for a special blessing on them right now, that they would know they are wanted and accepted. We sing

32

praises to you, as Mary did, upon the knowledge of Your great work! We stand in your presence, anticipating Your perfect will in our lives... Lord, we have trusted You with the size of our family, and You have chosen to place this child in the womb, we ask for Your wisdom to guide and show us how to properly oversee this life that You have given us. PRAISE YOU GOD! In Jesus' name, Amen!

The Beginning of Life

It is so important to realize the capability of your child, from the moment they are conceived. God knits the child within you, and has given them a spirit of their own. At what point does that spirit become viable? At what point can they feel and detect your love or your rejection? Some are now suggesting from the moment life begins as a single cell. I would like to encourage you, then, to be on your guard against negative thoughts and feelings toward your baby, and do all that you can to being to pray for them, speak to them, and bond with them right from the start. Our goal should be to establish an immediate bond with the baby through prayer, thanksgiving, meditation, and lifestyle.

According to Van den Bergh, B. R. H., chronic maternal anxiety directly correlates with fetal behavior, suggesting the need to be anxious for nothing (Phil 4:6). Remember Job, who was patient in all things, blessing the Lord regardless of his circumstances? It would be my prayer for you that you might find peace during your early prenatal days, overcoming all struggles in the name of Jesus Christ.

Spend your time dreaming of all the things the Lord is about to give you, and of all the things you are going to share with your child. It is very humbling to realize that part of you is going to live within this child for the rest of their life, based on what part of "you" is given to them. See to it that you give them your very best, knowing that you are not perfect, but that you desire to pass along your strengths.

Did you know that the prenatal period is a very sensitive time in your child's life, where opportunities exist to enhance their ability to form relationships? It is also a time rich in learning, and parents can take advantage of many techniques to ensure their child reaches their full human potential intellectually, emotionally, and physically. Mind, body, and spirit can be nurtured from conception through 40 weeks given the right stimulation from the parents.

Pregnancy is not a grace period free of consequences before birth. Pregnancy is the ultimate period of opportunity for parents to create fully loved, fully formed babies who are truly prepared to live a good life and create a better world. Dr. David B. Chamerlain

Quiet Moment

- Tell your baby that you love them, either out loud or in spirit
- Tell your baby that you want them and accept them
- Promise your baby that you will give them the best possible start to life
- Realize that your baby will have love for you, even from the womb
- Remember your baby is affected by the biochemicals of your emotions
- Give your baby a triple hug - in the mind by communicating something loving to them, in body by rocking them, and in spirit by praying for them and worshipping with them. Don't let shyness prevent you from expressing the love your baby needs!

When Is The Due Date?

You can use this chart to get an estimated day of delivery. The actual length of pregnancy is an average of 38 weeks, but because it is difficult to know exactly when a woman ovulates, the medical community has added the first two weeks prior to ovulation to make a total of 40 weeks. So, if you conceived three weeks ago, you will be considered five weeks pregnant according to the 40 week pregnancy scale. Keep in mind, a normal pregnancy is from 38 weeks until 42 weeks. Although 42 weeks would be uncomfortable, it is still within the normal limits and safe provided the baby and placenta are doing well.

How to calculate a due date

An average pregnancy lasts 280 days or 40 weeks -- starting with the first day of the last normal menstrual period (LMP) as day one. An estimated date of delivery (EDD) can be calculated by calculating the following:

1. Determine the first day of your last menstrual period.
2. Count back three calendar months from that date.
3. Add one year and seven days to that date.

This method of determining your due date is based off of the Näegele's Rule, which uses the 28-day menstrual cycle as a basis. Dates may have to be adjusted if your cycle is different. Keep in mind that less than 10 percent of women actually deliver on the baby's due date.

Who Will You Choose For A Provider?

This might be your single-most important decision you make on your journey to parenthood. Truly, who you choose to deliver your child ought to be considered as heavily as how you choose what church you want to fellowship with. If your provider is not compatible with your beliefs, you are in for a world of strife. It is important to start learning all you can about the process of birth so that you know what you would like from your care provider. Here are some questions to ask yourself:

- Do you want a natural birth?
- Do you want to take an active role in the decision-making process?
- Where do you want to be when you deliver your baby?
- Do you want a provider who a Christian?
- Do you want a doctor or a midwife?
- Do you want a doula?
- Is your provider accepting of alternative methods of giving birth?
- Who is an approved provider in your insurance plan?
- Are you willing to spend extra money to have the birth you want if no one in your insurance plan is willing to help you in the manner of birth you would like?
- Do you want your provider to attend the majority of your labor or are you okay with them showing up at the end when it is time to deliver the baby?
- Do you want a specific person to be at your birth or are you okay with an on-call staff of providers?
- What kinds of alternative birthing options are available at the location where you choose to deliver?
- Are you choosing the hospital with the NICU out of fear of the unknown and are you willing to trust in birth, regardless of where you deliver?

- Are you looking for a provider who has experience with a "hands-off" style of management of labor and delivery?
- Many have not been trained in how to help a woman have a natural birth… Do they know how to help you achieve this?

It might seem a little early to be thinking about these things right now, but if you settle in to a provider that you later find out does not support your ideals, it is awful hard to change later in pregnancy, though not impossible. Be a good steward of making the decision of who will be a steward over you. This decision is paramount!

Father, we ask right now that you guide us to the right provider, and that you would make it perfectly apparent that it is they who You have chosen for us. Lord, make it totally obvious to us who You would like us to employ. May they be of one mind and one accord with us, Lord. Open that door for us in Your timing, in Jesus name, Amen.

Pregnancy Dedication

Many Christians will publicly hold a baby dedication after the birth to announce before God and family that they are dedicated to raising the baby in the ways of the Lord. I would like to propose that you hold a "pregnancy" dedication, promising the Lord publicly that you will do all that you can to be a good hostess for your baby's development.

Redeemer, we stand on your grace and present this precious child to you, dedicating their life to you. We commit them to your care, and ask that you strengthen us and equip us as parents so that we can train them up in Your ways. Rabbi, teach us how to be healthy in all ways in order to give this child the best start possible. We present this life within to You now, asking that they would be the child of God that you have called them to be. In Jesus' name, Amen.

You can keep this as a simple prayer, have a get-together at your home, or even be bold enough to hold a pregnancy dedication at your church. Why not?

Bible Study Discussion

1. Was your baby planned or a surprise?

2. Do you feel a bond with the baby yet?

3. What dreams have you been having about the baby?

4. When is your due date?

5. What part of this chapter stands out to you?

Chapter Three
The Joys of Pregnancy

This could possibly be the most miraculous time in your life, as your body makes incredible changes to sustain the new life within you. Fathers, too, will be going through some wonderful heart changes as they set their mind and spirit for parenthood. Many a couple has complained about some of the changes, however, here is your chance to shine as a grateful child of God. You can begin to practice the miracle of joy in all situations, even in the minor discomforts of pregnancy. Guard your hearts and minds fiercely during this tender time of change.

Wonderful Changes in Her:

Ω Fatigue
Ω Breast tenderness & enlargement
Ω Pelvic cramping/discomfort
Ω Nausea/vomiting
Ω Moodiness
Ω Constipation
Ω Hormones
Ω Urinary frequency
Ω Headaches & dizziness
Ω Weight gain
Ω Back pain
Ω Swollen ankles
Ω Vivid dreams

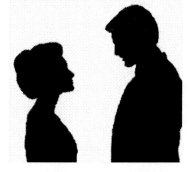

Wonderful Changes in Him:

Ω A new sense of responsibility
Ω Worry about provision
Ω Insomnia
Ω Fatigue
Ω Sympathy symptoms
Ω A need to protect her

Ω A new sense of patience!

<u>Dealing with the changes</u>

First Trimester

Ω Fatigue

You may need up to 12 hours of sleep each night, so make sure that you go to bed early enough. If you nap, research shows that the most restful naps are either twenty minute naps, or two hour naps. If you cannot get two hours, then make it for twenty minutes and get up. You may also want to make sure that you are getting adequate nutrition, especially iron. Don't forget your prenatal vitamin, and avoid soft drinks and sugar snacks.

Ω Breast tenderness & enlargement

Try using a support bra made with 100% cotton. If your breasts are making you uncomfortable at night, try wearing a bra to bed. Avoid under-wire bras from here on out, as they put pressure on tender milk ducts and can cause infection after breast feeding has begun. The areolas (pigmented area around the nipples) will enlarge, darken, and may become covered in small bumps called Montgomery's tubercles (enlarged sweat glands). The veins become more prominent and may be darker in color.

Ω Pelvic cramping/discomfort

During the first trimester, they pregnancy is sustained by the hormone progesterone, which is secreted by a small ovarian cyst called the corpus leutum. Once the placenta is fully functional at the beginning of the second trimester, this small cyst may be the source of some pelvic pain, usually on the side. Also, menstrual-like cramps are normal as well.

Ω Nausea/vomiting

It is thought that hormonal changes is the cause of "morning sickness" which can actually occur any time of day. Gastrointestinal changes may also play a role, as the stomach empties more slowly. Eat a piece of toast or crackers in the morning before getting up. Ginger has been a popular remedy, and many add this to a caffeine-free tea. Avoid over the counter or prescription medication if possible, as no medication is 100% safe.

Ω Moodiness

Although hormones can wreak havoc on your emotions, you don't have to give in to temptation to lose all countenance. Sometimes it is good to talk about how you are feeling with your loved ones, to get it off your chest. Pregnancy is not an excuse to behave rude or unbecomingly, yet it is understandable that you may be out of sorts for a time. Lift your hands in faith during these times of trial, and stand strong against any tendency to lose control. You *can* do all things through Christ who strengthens you!

Ω Constipation

Throughout pregnancy, the bowels begin to slow down and become sluggish. Whatever you do, don't take a chemical laxative, it can cause a miscarriage. Try drinking plenty of water, and eating a balanced diet high in fiber.

Ω Hormones

Progesterone and Estrogen are increasing at amazing rates during early pregnancy, which can be responsible for many of these changes you are experiencing.

Ω Urinary frequency

Because you are drinking more water, you will be using the ladies room more. Additionally, your growing uterus is pressing against the bladder, lessening the amount of volume it can hold, requiring you to empty it more frequently.

Ω Headaches & dizziness

Again, it is important to think twice prior to taking any over-the-counter medication for minor discomforts. Avoid undue amounts of stress, dehydration, lack of sleep, or low blood sugar (hunger).

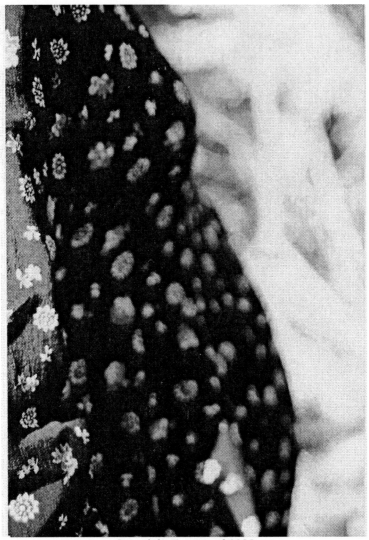

Copyright Townsend 1998

Ω Weight gain

Although some women lose weight in the first trimester, pregnancy is no time to diet. Keeping in mind that each woman is different, the normal weight gain for pregnancy is 25 to 30 pounds overall. Consult your care provider for the right amount of weight gain for you.

How The Baby Grows

Life begins at conception, and the mystery of the spiritual capabilities of this little child is just now being explored. Scientists are now looking at cellular memory, suggesting that even the first experiences in life make an impression on who this person will be. It is very important to respect every action that is taken to make sure the baby thrives from the start. Here are some of the milestones that your child wants to share with you. At the end of each chart, write a love note to your baby to give them when they are older…

Week 1-2	To make things consistent, medical professionals measure pregnancy from the first day of your last menstrual period. *You are not actually pregnant at this time.* Your overall health will play an important role in the baby's development.
Week 3	Conception has taken place and life begins. At conception, the gender is determined. The Lord knows this child by name, and loves him/her more than we can ever know!
Week 4	Implantation occurs! The baby will burrow itself into the lining of the uterus, perhaps loosening a little menstrual flow just before you would expect your normal period. This is normal, yet not all women experience spotting.
Week 5	Your baby now has three layers! The ectoderm, which will later develop into the nervous system, the mesoderm (middle layer) which will develop into the heart, bones, muscles, kidneys, and reproductive system, and the endoderm, a simple tube, will develop into the intestines, liver, pancreas, & bladder.
Week 6	What a difference a week makes! The heart now begins to beat! Baby is now an embryo and is about 1/17 of an inch long. Major growth will take place this week, as the eyes and ears begin to form, the umbilical cord is growing, most organs are being formed, and buds from the body appear that will become the arms and legs.

Week 7	Mommy, look at me! I am almost as big as a grain of rice! See how smart I am? My brain is really growing fast, and my eyes have lenses, my nose is getting nostrils, my tummy is growing intestines, I am getting a pancreas and bronchi for my lungs. My arms and legs are getting bigger and pretty soon my fingers and toes will start taking shape.
Week 8	Guess what Mom and Dad. I am starting to grow teeth in my gums, and if you take my ultrasound picture, you might even see my heart fluttering. You should see my feet! They are starting to get notches for toes and I even have elbows on my arms. Thanks for feeding me with really good food to make me very strong!
Week 9	My eyes are taking shape and now I am getting a tongue. If you look really close, you'll even see that my bones are starting to form. I need lots of protein and calcium Mom.
Week 10	Watch me move! Now I can swim around, but even though my joints are almost all done forming, you can't feel me yet. But soon you will!
Week 11	You're not going to believe this, but I am going to grow one inch this week! Yep! My head is half of my length, my eyes are fusing shut, and my irises are starting to form. Sometime this week or next, my blood is going to start circulating between me and my placenta. Pretty cool, huh?
Week 12	Yep, now I have fingers and toes, and now I am getting hair and fingernails. My gender begins to develop more, and almost all of my organs are formed, but will still be growing throughout pregnancy. My kidneys are working and there is more and more amniotic fluid to swim in!
Mom & Dad's Love Note	

Love Notes (Con't)

Ω Leg Cramps

Many women experience leg cramps due to a deficiency of calcium in their diet. The answer is simple – increase the intake of calcium. During a cramp, the discomfort can be relieved by lifting the toes and foot as high as possible, lowering the heel of the foot, and stretching the calf muscle until the cramp stops.

Ω Round Ligament Pain

It is often of great concern to many women to experience pain in the lower abdomen and groin. As the uterus grows, the ligaments that hold it in place begin to stretch, and may cause pain in some women. One of these ligaments are attached to the sacrum in the back, causing a dull aching pain in the lower back/buttocks. Other areas of ligament discomfort are in the front of the pelvis along the bikini line. These short stabbing or dull pains should only last a few moments and be of little concern. If stabbing pain persists, contact your care provider.

Unfortunately, there is little that can be done to alleviate round ligament pain. Use these small aches and pains to practice your breathing and relaxing skills in preparation for labor. It is good to get into the habit of responding to pain not by tensing up, but rather by releasing your muscles and tension as you combat it with abdominal breathing.

Ω Constipation

The change in hormone levels during pregnancy affects the function of the digestive system, slowing it down. In addition, a growing baby puts pressure on the bowel, which with the two combined, can lead to constipation. Keep drinking plenty of water (eight glasses a day is best), eat more fiber, prunes, salad, and other roughage. Alfalfa tablets have been useful for some women, providing extra roughage needed. Make sure to get mild exercise, as this helps to keep things moving along. Again, do not take over the counter laxatives.

Ω Hemorrhoids

One of the many marks of motherhood is the experience with hemorrhoids. Not all women get them, but it is a very common problem. Hemorrhoids are basically varicose veins that have developed due to increased pressure in that area.

Warm baths may relieve the discomfort, and many women have found relief with witch hazel compresses. Avoiding long periods of standing will also help, as standing for extended amounts of time can cause your circulation to become sluggish and worsen the problem. Avoid straining during a bowel movement, as this is the primary cause of the problem.

The design of the American toilet could very well be the culprit in many hemorrhoid problems in our country. European and Asian countries provide toilets that allow a person to actually squat while having a bowel movement. Squatting is the natural position assumed by many toddlers as they "do their business" in the middle of their play time. There is something about squatting vs. sitting that relieves the pressure that causes hemorrhoids. This is a another indication that squatting during birth is better on the bowel than sitting...

It may be next to impossible, and dangerous for a pregnant woman to squat on a toilet, so the next best thing is to set a step stool in front of the toilet to elevate the legs in a "mock-squat." Women notice that they strain less, as this also helps with constipation.

Week 13	So I have been working on my vocal chords, my eyes are getting closer together, my ears are going to the right spot, and my organs are starting to practice.
Week 14	I am really getting big, 'cause I am 3 ½ inches and I weigh about 1-2 ounces. Since my fingers and hands can move, I have been trying to see how they work. Oh, and guess what. My placenta that I have been working on started functioning this week!
Week 15	I don't have much to report, except that my bones keep getting stronger, and you can see my veins through my skin. I have a little hair called lanugo all over me, but that will go away in about ten weeks or so. If you could

	see me, I'd show you how I can suck my thumb now. How have you been feeling, Mom?
Week 16	You know what? If you haven't already, you might be able to feel me move now. I might feel like wings of a fluttering butterfly on your tummy… If you don't feel me yet, don't worry, you will soon!
Week 17	I've been putting on weight, a little fat for padding, and my heart is really pumping now. I have been growing really fast, so I will need extra nourishment Mom. Thanks!
Week 18	I think I am almost about a half a pound now, and you might even feel me get the hiccups.
Week 19	It's been a while in this amniotic fluid, so I decided to make some vernix to coat my skin and keep it from getting too soggy. Will you promise to rub it into my skin like lotion after I'm born? It's really good for my skin…
Week 20	Where's the brush, 'cause I'm getting' hair! I am about 7 ½ inches long and almost one whole pound… Hey Mom, we're half-way there! Yippee!
Week 21	So I was thinking of slowing down my growing and start working on my organs, making sure they are working just right. What do you think? Lots of raw vegetables sounds good right now… maybe some grapes too...
Week 22	This week I'm gonna start growing my brain, so I'll need a lot of protein and brain food. My eyelids and eyebrows are done, and I am about a pound heavy. Moving right along!

Week 23	I am looking more and more like you each day, my proportions are getting better, and if I accidentally come out now, with some help, I just might survive... But I'd rather stay inside for a while longer...
Week 24	I've been working out, and my muscles are really pumping up! I just might get up to 1 1/3 of a pound by the end of the week. Are you proud of me?
Week 25	Look at my back, Mom. See my backbone? I'm really busy with that, God has really been doing it, but I am proud too. Thanks for helping me, Mom and Dad, by being healthy.
Week 26	God has really been fixing up my lungs, getting them ready for breathing. Also, my brain has been trying to do more brainwave activity for my visual and auditory systems. By the way, are you okay? I wanted to tell you that I love you so much!
Week 27	I am growing so much, I am about 9.5 inches, but more importantly, my brain is really growing and needs protein more and more. My eyelids are starting to open and the retina in my eyes are starting to grow too.
Mom & Dad's Love Note	

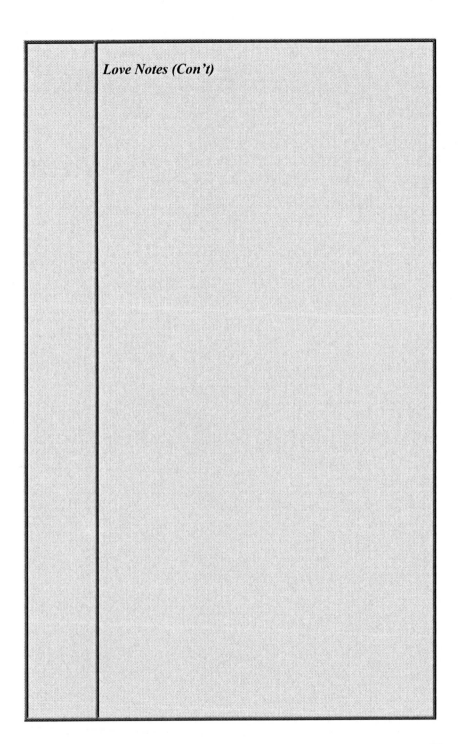

Love Notes (Con't)

Third Trimester

Ω Heartburn

As the baby grows and the uterus puts pressure on the stomach, it is normal for the food in the stomach to be pushed back into the esophagus, causing heartburn. This sometimes painful sensation in the middle of the chest can be alleviated by eating smaller, more frequent non-spicy or non-fried meals. Avoid over-the-counter medication for this issue, as some may interfere with mineral absorption.

Ω Painful Pelvic Joints

There is a hormone that is naturally secreted during pregnancy called relaxin. The purpose of this hormone is to relax the joints in the pelvis in order to make more room for the passage of the baby. As the joints begin to soften and relax, nerves can become pinched and the joints can actually separate. Proper body mechanics and posture can help alleviate this condition. For example, when turning over in bed, keep the knees together as you turn, preventing damage to the joint in your pubic bone (symphysis pubis).

Ω Braxton-Hicks Contractions

The uterus begins contracting long before labor begins as a way to exercise and prepare for birth. These contractions are different from true labor and do not open or change the cervix. The contractions can by rhythmic or intermittent, but will usually be relieved by changing your position or a tall glass of water. For some women, Braxton-hicks contractions can be painful. If this is the case, use the opportunity to practice your relaxation and coping skills to get a head start on labor!

Ω Discomfort During Sleep

It can get awful uncomfortable in the latter months in bed. The pressure placed on your body while laying down increase, and you must get a little creative to stay comfortable. While lying down, place a pillow between your legs to lift the upper leg enough so as not to put pressure on the hip. Also put a pillow under your arm to relieve the pressure on your shoulder. Do not lay on your back, as the weight of the baby will put pressure on the vena cava, a large vein between your uterus and spine, causing your blood pressure to dangerously drop.

Another position that many women like is to lie in a semi-stomach position. As you lay almost on your stomach, put the arm that is behind you straight against your back, and bring the other arm up at a 90 degree angle with a pillow underneath it. Keep the bottom leg straight, and bring the upper leg up to a 90 degree angle, with a pillow of support as well. This creates the fewest pressure points and is quite comfortable, even after you have had your baby. It also provides for good mechanics, as when it is time to turn over, you can keep the pillow between your knees and carry it over to the other side, allowing your knees to stay together and prevent a cartilage tear in the pubic bone.

Ω Swelling

It is quite normal to have some swelling of feet and ankles in the last weeks, especially if the third trimester is in the hot months. Spend some time every day with your feet elevated, avoiding long periods of standing.

It becomes a problem when your face becomes swollen as well. This may be an indication of pregnancy induced hypertension (toxemia) and requires immediate medical attention.

Week 28	You're not going to believe it, but my eyes are completely formed! But even better, I can hear you and recognize your voice! I love it when you sing and play with me...
Week 29	My head is now in proportion to my body, and my brain can now control simple breathing. I can see light, hear sound, taste and smell too.
Week 30	Yep, I'm almost 3 pounds now. That lanugo hair is starting to go away, I wonder what that means. My toes are growing nails, and my bone marrow is making red blood cells. Isn't God so great?
Week 31	So I am going to slow down growing for a little bit, and work on my brain again. God says eat extra protein again...

Week 32	Bet you can't guess how much I weigh… Okay, I'll tell you. Almost 4 pounds!!! You should see my hair grow. Or at least I think it's growing. I wonder how much I will have when I am born…
Week 33	Are you staying comfortable Mommy? I hope I am not taking up too much room. By the way, my skin isn't red anymore, now it is pink… I can't wait until we look into each other's eyes…
Week 34	I am learning to close my eyes while I am asleep, and open them when I am awake, just like you!
Week 35	If I am like many babies, then I am about five and a half pounds. It's starting to get a little tight in here. I've been thinking about what I like better, head up or head down… I can hear you better with my head up, but I was thinking down was good too…
Week 36	Ok, head down is probably the way to go. Sorry if my head gets in the way or gets uncomfortable. I've been putting on some fat, they say it makes a kid look cute… I'll still be gaining a lot of weight, about an ounce a day!
Week 37	A good 6.5 lbs, I am really getting ready for something, but I am not sure what yet. I've been copying your breathing movements… I really love you Mom, I hope you know that…
Week 38	I know your getting tired and uncomfortable, Mom. Me too, it's really tight in here, but I am growing so much each day, and it seems like being inside you would be the best if everything is normal. I still have a couple weeks yet, and that really isn't that long if you think about it.
Week 39	I am probably about seven pounds now, and I hope you don't mind, but I'd like to start thinking about coming out. Not sure when, but I'll let you know for sure when I am ready. Whatever you do, make sure that the time comes

	by itself unless something is really wrong. That is so much better for me, when it happens all by itself. And, it is more than likely going to be easier for you if we wait for it to happen by itself. You can do it, Mom, God will strengthen you…
Week 40!	Well, this is the week they said it would be, and maybe it is true, who knows? Hard to tell that for sure. Are you doing okay? I am so proud you are my Mom. I love you for loving me and making such good choices for me, even when it is hard for you. Thanks sooooo much! I can almost feel your warm arms around me.
Week 41	Don't worry Mom. If I am still inside, it is because I need to be for some reason. This happens a lot, and is still in the normal range. If everything is okay, then I will wait if you will. Don't be scared, God is taking care of us.
Week 42	Mom, I'll give you a scripture. *They that wait upon the Lord will renew their strength, they will soar on wings like eagles, they will run and not grow wary, they will walk and not be faint.* *Isaiah 40:31*
Mom & Dad's Love Note	

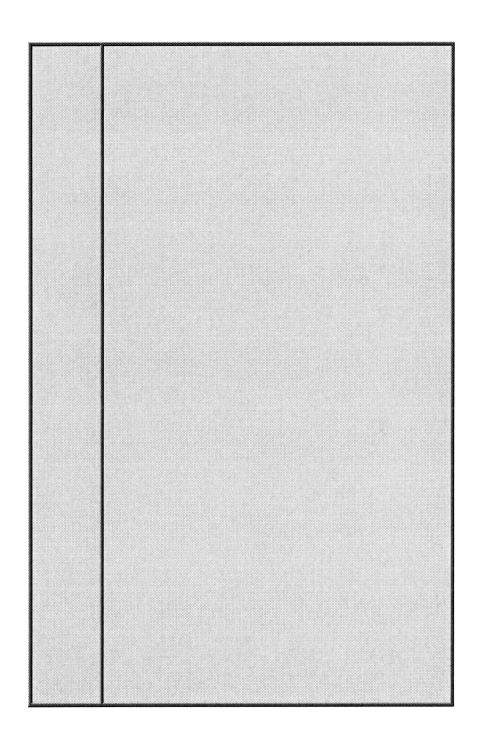

Bible Study Discussion

1. What discomforts are you experiencing right now?

2. What are you doing to alleviate them?

3. How are you keeping a positive outlook?

4. How can you represent Christ when you talk about your discomforts to others?

5. What part of this chapter stands out to you?

Chapter Four
Building A Temple

Truly, He is the Lord of all creation, and He dwells within us. We get the blessed privilege to assist the Lord in building one of His little children while we carry them for nine months. The Bible tells us that our bodies are the temple of God, and we can honor Him by treating them with respect. We do this by not smoking, by not taking drugs, by not engaging in illicit sex, by exercising appropriately, and by nourishing our body with good, wholesome food. Although we may desire to engage in unhealthy habits, we abstain and offer our body up as a "living sacrifice" that would be holy and acceptable to God.

We understand that our body is a temple of the Lord, and we realize the very tiny baby that we hold within us will grow into a beautiful temple as well. This little child is as dependant upon God to knit him in the womb as he is dependant upon us to nourish him in a proper way that would insure his solid health.

If we choose the Standard American Diet (SAD), however, he is certainly off to a less-than-ideal start. As America chooses a diet high in fat, simple carbohydrates, and refined sugar, she has sacrificed better nutrition to the god of convenience and is now paying the very dear price of heart disease, high rates of cancer and stroke.

We are what we eat, so every bite that crosses our lips should be of high nutritional value, wholesome, and beneficial to the child. This chapter will offer nutritional guidelines as well as outline how to make simple changes in the diet that can have far-reaching and long-term benefits for our babies. Change doesn't always come easy, so we take one step at a time as we walk the narrow path that leads to solid health. We certainly do not eat to get spiritually closer to God (1 Cor 8:1), but we do it as a way to honor Him and to show Him that we desire to have His little temple constructed out of the good stuff!

Basic Nutritional Needs

This book will cover the very basics of nutritional needs of the pregnant mother and her baby. For a more in-depth look at nutrition and pregnancy, read *The Naturally Healthy Pregnancy: The Essential Guide to Nutritional and Botanical Medicine for the Childbearing Years* by Shonda Parker. Also, please look into the Brewer Diet at www.blueribbonbaby.org and www.birthingnaturally.net for great resources.

According to Dr. Brewer, a poor nutritional diet can cause many problems in both the baby and the mother during pregnancy. If a mother eats poorly, she runs the risk of having a low birth weight or premature baby, a brain damaged baby with lowered intelligence, a hyperactive baby with irritability, an infection-prone baby with more illnesses, and even a stillborn baby. She also stands the chance of metabolic toxemia of late pregnancy, anemia, premature detachment of the placenta (abruptio placenta), infections of the lungs, kidneys, and liver, and a more difficult labor & delivery.

Remember: It is not healthy for you and your unborn baby to go even 24 hours without good food! - Dr. Brewer

Protein

Protein is the building block of tissue. The normal pregnancy diet requires 80 - 100 grams of protein each day, and beyond 100 grams if you are high-risk or carrying twins. The following is a chart that lists the amount of protein in various foods. Certainly animal products are the highest in protein and you can see that it would not be very difficult to achieve the recommended daily allowance. It is possible to consume too much protein during pregnancy, so keep track of what you are eating and get a feel for how much is enough. If you choose a vegetarian diet, you can see that it will take a little more effort to reach the RDA as well as ensure a complete protein, but it is certainly not impossible.

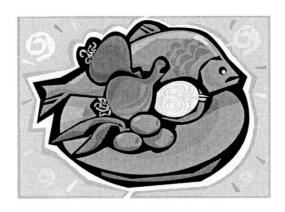

Food	Portion Size	Protein (Grams)
Beans, refried	1 cup	16
Bread	1 slice	3
Beef, round roast	3 oz	25
Broccoli	½ cup	3
Cheese (any variety)	1 oz	8
Chicken, white meat	3.5 oz	31
Cottage Cheese	½ cup	14
Egg (Whole)	1	6
Frankfurter	2 oz	7
Halibut	3 oz	18
Milk (Skim, Whole)	1 cup	8
Milk (2%)	1 cup	12
Pasta	1 cup	5
Peanut Butter	1 Tbsp	4
Rice (brown, cooked)	1 cup	5
Tofu	100 grams	9
Tuna in oil	3 oz	24
Turkey, light	3 oz	28
Yogurt	1 cup	8

What Does Protein Consist Of?

Protein is an organic compound that consists of carbon, oxygen, hydrogen, and nitrogen. It is responsible for synthesizing some of the structures of the body such as muscle and anabolic hormone activity. Your baby's body will need protein for basic growth, as well as for many of the major biological functions. Perhaps when the Bible speaks of how God knits us together in the womb, He was speaking of protein!

Protein consists of 22 amino acids, considered the building blocks of life. There are two types of amino acids, essential and non-essential. There are nine essential amino acids, which cannot be produced by the human body, and therefore need to be consumed by food.

For each protein, there are specific amino acids in a specific amount. Some combinations of amino acids make up a complete protein; others do not. For a protein to be considered complete, it must contain all of the 9 essential amino acids. If a protein is lacking one or more of the essential acids, we can compensate by eating another food in combination to make a complete protein.

Complete proteins come from animal sources such as fish, dairy, chicken, beef, and eggs. Protein from plant sources is incomplete, and needs to be combined with a complimentary food that contains the missing essential amino acids. Examples of plant combinations include rice and beans, cereal and milk, beans and corn, bread and cheese.

Essential Amino Acids	Non-essential Amino Acids
Histidine	Alanine
Isoleucine	Arginine
Leucine	Asparagine
Lysine	Aspartate
Methionine	Cysteine
Phenylalanine	Glutamate
Threonine	Glutamine
Tryptophan	Glycine
Valine	Proline
	Serine
	Tyrosine

Iron

Iron is an essential component of your red blood cells, and it is responsible for carrying oxygen throughout your body. Oxygen, of course, is vitally important for the health of the fetus. When we become deficient in iron, we have what is called anemia. Anemia can cause fatigue, dizziness, and rapid heart rate, as well as compromise the benefit of oxygen to the baby. It is common for the average expecting American woman to be deficient in iron. For this reason, we need to be determined to eat the foods that are rich in this nutrient not only for the benefit of our child, but also for our own well-being.

Foods that are high in Iron:

Red Meat	Clams
Turkey	Shrimp
Sardines	Pumpkin Seeds
Spinach	Raisins
Nuts	Molasses
Fortified Cereal	Brewers Yeast

Folic Acid

Sometimes called Folate, folic acid is a B vitamin which is is an important nutrient that helps prevent birth defects. Many women don't realize that it is important to take folic acid *before* they conceive to create the healthiest environment for the baby before they take up residence in the womb. Birth defects such as spina bifida and anencephaly (severe underdevelopment of the brain) occur during the first 28 days of life in the womb – usually before a woman even knows that she is pregnant.

Make it a goal to get at least 400 micrograms per day during early pregnancy to reduce the risk of birth defects. Folic acid is found in:

- Green vegetables like kale and spinach
- Orange juice
- Enriched grains like cereals, breads, rice, and pastas
- Prenatal vitamin supplements

What to Strive For

Much of the food that is eaten is over-processed and low in nutrient value. Don't sell out to the god of convenience and prepare meals for your baby that are devoid of any real nutritive substance.

"And God said, Behold, I have given you every herb bearing seed, which is upon the face of all the Earth, and every tree, in the which is the fruit of a tree yielding seed; to you it shall be for food."
Genesis 1:29

Whenever possible, eat food in it's original state – whole food. God's provision is good, and the food He created is made to nourish our bodies. It is when we break it down, dehydrate it, change it, refine it, package it, etc. that it becomes less than healthy. Eating raw, original food maximizes the potential for nutrient availability.

Whole Food	Changed Food
Whole Wheat Kernels	White Bread/Pasta
Brown Rice	White rice
Steak (Beef, Chicken, Fish)	Lunchmeat/Pepperoni
Fresh Fruit	Canned Fruit
Whole Milk	2% Milk/Yogurt/Cheese
Tomatoes	Ketchup
Oatmeal	Cheerios

It is not necessary to remove changed food from your diet, however the majority of what you eat should be in its original form. Evaluate each bite you take to see if it is a whole food, ensuring that the main percentage of your diet that is made up of whole foods.

Enzymes

Living enzymes exist in uncooked, un-pasteurized food. They are important for the digestion and absorption of nutrients, they give you energy, and perhaps play a far more significant role than we ever imagined. Science is now exploring the possibility that enzymes have quantum characteristics, meaning that the information contained within the cell is not bound there, but can be communicated amongst other cells.[1]

This might suggest that the living food you eat (Meaning the enzymes haven't been destroyed by heat or pasteurization) have the capability to move throughout your body in cooperation with the information from other cells and provide restoration and healing. This information is on the frontier of science, yet makes perfect Biblical sense. God gave us living food, every plant bearing seed, to nourish our bodies. Make living food a majority of the food that you eat!

What to Avoid

Monosodium Glutamate (MSG)

MSG is a flavor enhancer that is in just about every pre-packaged food available. It allows food manufacturers to use lower quality, poorer tasting food and pass it off as flavorful. Most know that MSG is in Chinese food, but look at some surprising sources for this very unhealthy additive:

- Ranch dressing
- Chicken noodle soup
- Most broths
- Flavored snack chips
- Chili
- Sausage
- Packaged meals
- Microwave meals
- Raviolis
- Macaroni & cheese
- Breading on fish, chicken, etc.
- Flavoring on grilled, skinless chicken breasts
- Just about anything that is preserved

Now that people are becoming more aware of MSG, the food industry has found new ways to disguise MSG in the label. If you see hydrolyzed _____ protein (fill in the blank with soy, vegetable, corn, etc), or natural flavorings, then it contains MSG. There isn't much out there that does not have it... It really isn't good for you or your baby. It can cause birth defects and neurological damage to you both if used in excess.

Microwave

It is well known that using a microwave will alter the nutritive and protective qualities of breast milk, and therefore is greatly discouraged. You might want to ask yourself, "if it can alter the beneficial properties in milk, then can it do that to other foods?" If it isn't safe for your baby, then it isn't safe for you to eat either. Getting used to preparing food the old-fashioned way is a fun chore (but not impossible) especially if your motivation is out of love for your baby. If you cannot avoid it, then limit the amount of food you eat that is cooked or warmed by the microwave.

Citric Acid

Many people do not realize what citric acid is made from. If a Google search is conducted using the search terms "fermentation industry" and "citric acid," the source of this preservative is presented.

Bacteria and mold oppose and feed off each other. Most food is in danger of spoiling because of bacteria overgrowth, and one way to reduce this problem is to introduce mold into the food in a washed state. Thus, citric acid. The mold Aspergillus is grown by fermenting a raw material like lemons or molasses, then harvesting the mold by scraping off the top layer, rinsing and treating it, and then adding it to preserved food and beverages like soda.

I encourage you to start paying attention to the food that contains mold in the form of citric acid. I would also encourage you to do a little research regarding the mold Aspergillus, perhaps beginning with www.mold-help.org. Once you find out about this toxic black mold that is being put into your food, you might not want to consume it.

Fungal Toxins

Speaking of mold, you will want to make sure your environment is free from it. Stachybotrys is capable of taking a newborn's life if it is in your environment in large quantities.[2] Learn more about Stachybotrys and other dangerous molds that can be harmful to you and your family.

1. The DNA-wave Biocomputer Peter P. Gariaev, Boris I. Birshtein, Alexander M. Iarochenko, Peter J. Marcer, George G. Tertishny, Katherine A. Leonova, Uwe Kaempf
2. Clinical profile of 30 infants with acute pulmonary hemorrhage in Cleveland. Pediatrics. 2002 Sep; 110 (3): 627-37 Dearborn DG, Smith PG, Dahms BB, Allan TM, Sorenson WG, Montana E, Etzel RA.

Quiet Moment:

What can you eat today that will show your baby that you love them? Write down food you eat today for your baby to show them that you care about their body, and how you desire them to get a healthy start...

Things I ate for you today, honey...

Item _____ Date

Item _____ Date

Item _____ Date

Item _____ Date

Item _____ Date

Item _____ Date

Item _____ Date

Item _____ Date

Bible Study Discussion

1. Do you eat living food on a regular basis?

2. How do you want to change your diet?

3. Share with the group local resources for healthy food.

4. List everything you have eaten today. Did you get your recommended daily allowance?

5. What part of this chapter stands out to you?

Chapter Five
Pregnancy: It's A God Thing

There are many things in life that a skeptic could explain as coincidence, but when the events of pregnancy are compared to certain events in the Bible, it becomes unmistakably clear that God has indeed imprinted his signature into the female body. The miracle of pregnancy goes far beyond the testimony of creation, for hidden within the knitted fabric of gestational life, is the plan for salvation and the fingerprint of Jesus Christ Himself!

Zola Levitt, a messianic Jew, was given fantastic insight into the process of pregnancy and how it relates to the seven feasts of Israel, found in Leviticus - chapter twenty-three. He was able to see the plan of salvation written into the code of pregnancy, and you can obtain a wonderful video called "A Child Is Born" detailing this plan. For those interested, the video can be ordered at www.levitt.com.

In this book, we will look at how the Jewish feasts and observances of the Old Testament correlate with the growth of the Christian walk, as it relates to gestation. You will notice that from the time of the first observance, (the preparation for the Passover) to the time of the last feast, (the Feast of Dedication - Hanukkah), the exact amount of time it takes for normal pregnancy to be completed exists.

Along the way are preordained and scheduled feasts that coincide perfectly with certain events of pregnancy that paint a picture of God's plan for the Christian. Come explore how the seven feasts of Israel recorded in the book of Leviticus, combined with other Biblical observances, coincide exactly with the significant events of pregnancy, and how this points the way to eternal life!

Whenever a child is born in this world, he has already celebrated in a secret and divine way, the seven feasts of Israel.
– Zola Levitt

The Hebrew live by a 28-day lunar calendar, with the new moon marking the first day of the month. The first month of the year is not in January, as Western culture's sun-driven calendar begins, but on the first new moon of Spring. The did not have modern technology to dictate what month would mark Spring, so God gave them a wonderful sign. The almond tree would blossom at the end of winter, before the rest of the fruit trees. God's children knew that when they saw the blossoms on the almond tree, Spring was right around the corner. The next new moon would mark their "new year's day."

Appointed Days & The Feasts – According to Leviticus 23

Nissan	1st month in Jewish Calendar (Mar/Apr)
Lamb Selection Day	10th day of the first month
Passover	14th day of the first month
Unleavened Bread	15th day of the first month
First Fruits	Following Sunday
Feast of Weeks	50 days from First Fruits / Pentecost
Feast of Trumpets	1st day of the seventh month
Day of Atonement	10th day of the seventh month
Feast of Tabernacles	15th day of the seventh month
Hanukkah	280 days after Passover

Because all but one of these significant dates were determined by the phases of the moon and by the seasons, it could not be determined exactly which day they would fall on. As we celebrate Easter on Sunday every year, Passover can be any day of the week, depending on what day the full moon falls on. It is by this calendar and program that the Lord has imbedded His secret plan for the life of the Christian, made known to us through Jesus Christ. The following are the appointed days, feasts, the events of pregnancy, and how they relate with your growth in Christ; ultimately leading to eternal life:

THE DAY OF PREPARATION (PALM SUNDAY)
~ PRE-CONCEPTION

The LORD said to Moses and Aaron in Egypt, "This month is to be for you the first month, the first month of your year. Tell the whole community of Israel that on the tenth day of this month each man is to take a lamb for his family, one for each household. Exodus 12:1-3

The day of preparation happened four days prior to Passover, when the Hebrew family was to choose a perfect lamb that would be slaughtered at twilight on the fourteenth day of the first month, which was Passover. It is interesting that Jesus rode a donkey into Jerusalem on the tenth day of the first month, the day the Jews would "choose" a lamb, the day Christians celebrate as Palm Sunday.

It is also interesting that this happened on the tenth day, as the number ten represents the number of the law. There were ten commandments given to Moses in the desert, which would become the foundation of Hebrew living. They were a light that was shed on the nature of man, an honest look at the fact that we have a sinful nature, and that there must be some sort of standard to live by if we were to be of higher intelligence and capability. We needed the law to illuminate the fact that although God made us in Him image, we were still prone to wander and sin, and needed the commandments as a guidebook, so-to-speak, to live by. It is important to note that the law, in and of itself, cannot save us, for all have sinned and fallen short of the glory of God. None of us is righteous, and no one can keep every point of the law, all of the time. Yes, the law, the ten commandments, were a preparation for the heart of God's children. They were to point to our need of a Savior.

Growth In Christ:

You did not choose me, but I chose you and appointed you to go and bear fruit - fruit that will last. This is my command: Love each other. John 15:16-17

When a baby girl is born, all of the ovum (the eggs in her ovaries) are complete and formed. Whereas sperm is not formed until a day or so before it is released, the ovum have been selected long before they will every be fertilized and grown into a person.

There are two very important points to this passage as it relates to the Christian. First, we need to realize that long before the Christian has conceived Christ in their heart, before conception of the born-again soul takes place, they have already been chosen by the Father to be a servant of the Lord. There is a purpose and a plan for them, to bear fruit in their life that would leave a legacy for those who come after them, and that the fruit of their love should last.

Secondly, I believe that God might be giving us a hint to His will in this passage. To those of you who will be studying this correlation between pregnancy, the Lord, and salvation, it is noteworthy to see that God has placed a clue here in the passage of John 15. This speaks of being chosen prior to your conversion to Christ - prior to conception of the spirit of your soul. However, look again at the scripture:

You did not choose me, but I chose you and appointed you to go and bear fruit - fruit that will last. This is my command: Love each other.

The time of preconception is important to the Lord, for He has given us a command written in the above passage concerning His choosing of us – that we are to love each other. He links preconception, if you will, to loving each other.

Could it be that the Lord would be encouraging us to make sure that before we become parents, before we conceive a child, we are truly in love? Could He be telling us that it is very important for the marriage to be firmly established before we embark on the journey to parenthood? It is an interesting correlation if one studies God's plan for the growth of the Christian, saying that even before we "knew" Him, even before we were alive in Christ, He chose us and commanded that we love each other.

Many parents that have conceived out of wedlock or soon after their honeymoon would be quick to give this important advice regarding the necessity for solid love before family grows. Make it a special point to be in the center of God's will, ensuring your marriage is on solid ground, and built upon the Rock.

There is a beautiful analogy that is fitting, regarding the strength of marriage. Sailors know that a rope that is made of two strands twisted around each other is inferior to the one with three strands. When the pressure is put on, the two-stranded rope will snap. The three-stranded rope, however, withstands the pressure.

If a husband and wife try to survive the work of marriage on their own, the pressure may very well cause them to snap, and a divorce soon follows. If, however, they invite Jesus Christ into the fabric of their union, if He is wound and woven between them, they will be stronger and able to withstand any pressure placed upon them.

Jesus Christ. Make Him the third member of your marriage!

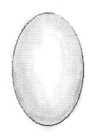

PASSOVER
~ OVULATION

The LORD's Passover begins at twilight on the fourteenth day of the first month. Leviticus 23:5

Successful fertilization begins with an ovum that is typically released on the fourteenth day of the first month of pregnancy. Similarly, Passover is observed on the fourteenth day of the first month of the Jewish year. It is celebrated in remembrance of the night in Egypt when God spared the firstborn son of any family who had applied the blood of the lamb (the one they chose on the tenth day of the month) upon the doorpost of their home, which ultimately led to their release from bondage. God "passed over" their homes because they had applied the blood to the door at the top, and on each side.

They took a branch of hyssop and dipped it into the blood of the sacrificed lamb that was in the basin at the threshold of the door. This is one of the Old Testament pictures of Christ, as the blood at the top, the sides, and in the basin at the bottom for the shape of – a cross!

Passover is a beautiful depiction of the crucifixion, as it speaks of that lamb that was sacrificed for the cleansing of sins. During the Passover dinner, a piece of matzoh bread is broken into three pieces. The middle piece is wrapped in linen, the father hides it away, and then it is found again. It is not fully understood by the Jews where this custom came from, but for the Christian, it is a beautiful picture of how the Lord, the second member of the Trinity, was broken, hidden away after being wrapped in linen, and then rediscovered on the third day. Even more wonderful is the picture of matzoh itself. It is a striped flat bread that has been pierced. Isaiah 53:5 says that He was pierced for our transgressions, wounded for our iniquities, and by His stripes we are healed. God uses everything in the Old Testament to point to Jesus Christ. Amazing.

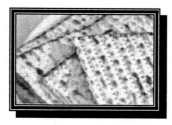

Parenthetically, Jewish tradition includes an egg on every Passover table. In most cultures, the egg represents new life. It is no surprise, then, that the egg on the Passover table represents the new life that they received apart from Egypt (Egypt has always been a symbol of worldliness). For this study, it is quite surprising and delightful that God chose this feast, of which they include the symbol of the egg on the table, to line up perfectly with the event of ovulation - the egg that literally is the chance for new life!

Growth In Christ:

The Bible says that while we were yet sinners, Christ died for us. Ovulation happens before life begins, it is correlated with Passover, and Passover is a symbol of the crucifixion, the sacrifice of the spotless Lamb, Jesus Christ, as He died for us on the cross. The ovulation of the egg now represents the sacrifice on the cross, while we were still "dead" in our transgressions. What a beautiful picture!

FEAST OF UNLEAVENED BREAD
~ FERTILIZATION

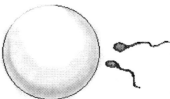

Once ovulation has taken place, fertilization must occur within 24 hours if it is to be successful. Look at the second feast of Israel.

On the fifteenth day of that month (one day after Passover) the LORD's Feast of Unleavened Bread begins; for seven days you must eat bread made without yeast. On the first day hold a sacred assembly and do no regular work. For seven days present an offering made to the LORD by fire. And on the seventh day hold a sacred assembly and do no regular work.' " Leviticus 23:6-8

After the children of Israel fled from Pharaoh and were wandering in the desert, God sent down from Heaven unleavened bread called manna (which means, "What is it?") which sustained them perfectly. This is why the feast of "unleavened bread" is celebrated. Jesus referred to himself as the "bread of life," and was without sin, which is pictured for us symbolically in the Bible as leaven. Jesus is our unleavened bread, was born in Bethlehem (which means "house of bread) and sustains us perfectly, even when we are in the deserts of life.

The feast of unleavened bread is the time when the seed is planted for the crop, signifying the promise of a harvest to come. How appropriate that this feast would happen at the right time, in synch with the implantation of the seed which promises a harvest, so-to-speak, of a new life nine months from now.

Growth In Christ:

In Genesis 12:7, God promised Abraham that unto his Seed he would give the land. Scholars, including the Apostle Paul in Galatians 3:16, conclude that this seed speaks of Jesus Christ. How perfect then is this picture, that once we accept Christ as Savior, once the Seed has penetrated the egg, we become a complete life form, ready to grow into a blessed child of God. Marvelous!

FEAST OF FIRST FRUITS
~ IMPLANTATION

The LORD said to Moses, "Speak to the Israelites and say to them: 'When you enter the land I am going to give you and you reap its harvest, bring to the priest a sheaf of the first grain your harvest. He is to wave the sheaf before the LORD so it will be accepted on your behalf; the priest is to wave it on the day after the Sabbath.
Leviticus 23:10-11

The new child travels down the fallopian tube at his own speed before he finds a comfortable place to implant. It might happen quickly or take many days. Just the same, the feast of First fruits is not on any specific timeline, except that it will happen on the Sunday after the feast of Unleavened Bread. It could take two days between the feast of Unleavened Bread and the Feast of First Fruits, or as many as six days. Because Unleavened Bread can happen at any day of the week, being determined by the phases of the moon, the distance between the two feasts can vary (just as the time it takes for implantation will vary). Regardless of what day Passover and Unleavened bread occur, First Fruits will always happen on the following Sunday. This allows for the timing of the new life to be his own, finding the blood of the womb at his own pace.

Growth In Christ:

The fallopian tubes are equipped with tiny microscopic hair, drawing the new life closer to the blood of the womb. After a person receives Christ, and is given new life in Him, he makes his way toward the knowledge of grace, that which is only given by the blood of Calvary. Indeed, Jesus does draw us near to Him, bringing us to the foot of the cross where the blood was shed. He desires us to know the great sacrifice that He made so that we might have life - life abundant.

Have you nestled into the reality of grace? Have you implanted into the nourishing fact that you are saved because of His sacrifice? Let the blood of grace nourish your soul as you grow into Him.

The baby grows the umbilical cord and placenta that attaches to the blood, the womb, in a beautiful picture of trust. In all of your ways, trust Him enough to grow your own cord of life into the essence of grace, which is the precious blood of Calvary leading to a new and resurrected life!

FEAST OF WEEKS - PENTECOST
~ RECOGNIZABLE HUMAN FETUS

'From the day after the Sabbath, the day you brought the sheaf of the wave offering, count off seven full weeks. Count off fifty days up to the day after the seventh Sabbath, and then present an offering of new grain to the LORD.' Leviticus 23:15-16

If you look at a growing embryo between the first day of life and the forty-ninth day of life, it is difficult to determine if it is an animal or a human. However, on the fiftieth day, it is now definitely recognizable as a human fetus. Obstetrical charts will have forty-nine pictures of daily development from conception onward, yet it is on the fiftieth day that experts agree this is an identifiable human - a "new" creature.

Interestingly, on the fiftieth day is the day of Pentecost, the day when the disciples received the Holy Spirit upon them, making them "new creatures" in Christ. They now had the promised Spirit of truth and were indeed born again.

Growth In Christ:

As the Christian has grown in grace, and accepted the blood of Calvary (the previous feast) as the only way of salvation, they understand the magnitude of God's mercy and the true meaning of salvation, which is His undying love and mercy for us. The only response to that, if one is truly sincere, is a total devotion to God, out of love and thankfulness to what He did. Truly, they have entered into the body of Christ, into the true church as a true born-again believer, a "new creature" in Christ.

Just as the fetus is unmistakably human at 50 days, when one observes the born-again at this stage in their life, they are more than obviously Christian! The evidence of their faith is seen in their actions, because truly they have allowed Christ to live within them. Their actions are those of service and love, repenting from their sinful ways and replacing that with charity and good works. Not because they have to, but because they want to let Christ manifest Himself through them, by the love that they demonstrate to others. Do people see Christ in you?

FEAST OF TRUMPETS
~ HEARING

The Lord said to Moses, "Say to the Israelites: 'On the first day of the seventh month you are to have a day of rest, a sacred assembly commemorated with trumpet blasts. Do no regular work, but present an offering made to the Lord by fire.'" Exodus 23:23-25

According to PG Hepper, the timeframe for the majority of fetuses to demonstrate the ability to respond to sound happens around the 30th week of pregnancy, or the 28th week of gestation. Human hearing has been shown to develop much earlier in controlled studies. However, in Biblical times, the evidence that the pregnancy was viable by the responsiveness of the baby to sound happened around this time in pregnancy. A loud noise or "trumpet blast" would create a startle response in the baby. This is fantastic because it correlates perfectly with the above scripture, which calls for a day of rest commemorated by the "sound" of trumpet blasts.

Growth In Christ:

In the Christian's walk, having been born again, a new kind of hearing will develop. The Christian will now be able to discern the voice of the Lord, which He uses in many ways. Non-believers often cannot understand when they hear a Christian say that "God told me _____" (fill in the blank). It is a foreign concept to them, because they have no spiritual ears. Of course, we do not usually hear audible voices, (although many in the Bible did, so it is not anti-scriptural if the Lord should speak audibly to you) but the Bible says that God will write His will upon the tablet of your heart (Psalm 40:8). It is with your heart that you begin to hear, as you grow in the Lord and get to know Him.

Secondarily, this feast focuses on the trumpet, which has significant implications for the Christian. The sound of the trumpet, in the scriptures, is a symbol of the rapture of the church (1 Corinthians 15). In our walk as a Christian, we know not when the Lord will return (Of that day or hour no man knows). There are many debates if it will happen before, during, or after the time of great tribulation. Regardless if we have just been saved, or have been walking with the Lord for over fifty years, we ought to be ready at any time, keeping our faces toward Heaven and our eyes on Jesus.

For the Lord Himself will come down from heaven, with a loud command, with the voice of the archangel, and with the trumpet call of God, and the dead in Christ will rise first. 1 Thessalonians 4:16

DAY OF ATONEMENT
~ HEMAGLOBIN A

The LORD said to Moses, "The tenth day of this seventh month is the Day of Atonement. Hold a sacred assembly and deny yourselves, and present an offering made to the LORD by fire. Do no work on that day, because it is the Day of Atonement, when atonement is made for you before the LORD your God. Anyone who does not deny himself on that day must be cut off from his people. I will destroy from among his people anyone who does any work on that day. You shall do no work at all. This is to be a lasting ordinance for the generations to come, wherever you live. It is a Sabbath of rest for your, and you must deny yourselves." Leviticus 23:26-32

Here, again, we see that number seven correlated with rest. May this be a time in your pregnancy for a Sabbath rest of sorts, your seventh month. Although we are blessed to be under grace and released from the curse of not keeping these feasts, they are a great picture of how the Lord has replaced them, especially this feast. It is not necessary to keep the feast of Atonement, because Christ has atoned for our sins now, so we are free from this ordinance. We celebrate the atonement even daily, praising God for His sacrifice. We can glean from these feasts however, and it is still important to refer to them to see what the Lord might teach us.

Perhaps the Lord is telling the young couple not to overdo it as they move into the third trimester. The second trimester, more than likely, was a time of energy and a sense of well-being. The third trimester, however, may be a little more taxing on the body. It is always good to take the advice of the Lord, and slow it down a little bit during the first week of your third trimester. Consider it a commemorative feast, dedicating this week to the Lord through a personal Sabbath. Sit back, kick your shoes off, and let others pamper you a little!

Beyond just a personal message, this feast is rich with spiritual implication regarding salvation and the unborn child. The baby is totally dependent on its mother for oxygen, however the oxygen that travels through the bloodstream is attached differently to the hemoglobin of the blood in young fetuses (hemoglobin F) and this type of fetal blood cannot sustain life outside the womb. Right about the 31-32 week of gestation (33-34 weeks of pregnancy), the hemoglobin begins to change to accommodate a more concentrated amount of oxygen and gradually becomes hemoglobin A, or adult blood.

In Leviticus 16, you can read about the day of Atonement, where the High Priest was to go into the Holy of Holies and present a blood sacrifice on behalf of the people. It is very interesting that this feast of the blood atonement falls at exactly the time the baby's blood is changing to a life-sustaining form.

The day of atonement was performed annually on the *tenth* day of the seventh month. The number ten, keep in mind, represents the law. On this day, the high priest would enter into the Most Holy Place of the Temple to offer ceremonial sacrifices for the forgiveness of the people. This is a direct picture of how Jesus Christ's blood was the all-sufficient, one-time sacrifice made on our behalf, so that we might be presented to the Lord as clean and washed of our sins.

Jesus entered into the throne room of God the Father to make atonement for all humanity once and for all, so that we need not repeat the process once a year, but daily take up our cross and follow Him! We are now no longer under the supervision of the law, (Galatians 3) but now are free to live by the Spirit of God. We have matured from child to co-heir with Christ, to receive the blessing of the Spirit of Jesus, growing ever closer to our "Abba-Father!" (Galatians 4).

We can do this because of the blood atonement of Jesus Christ, because of the blood he shed from seven places on his body. He was crushed for our iniquities, He denied Himself for our sake, therefore we then deny ourselves each and every day, crucify our fleshly desires, and live for Christ.

It is a difficult thing to do for one who is not close to the Lord, but when they understand the reason for the cross, they gladly deny themselves so that Christ might live through them. They desire to see God's will done on this Earth as it is in Heaven. We must put away the childish ways that we were once a slave to, and grow into the maturity that is required if we are going to live the effective Christian life.

Growth In Christ:

As this little baby is now able to sustain life outside the womb if necessary, so too is the Christian less dependent on the church to grow them. They begin to read the scriptures on their own, become more accountable to themselves and to God, and are capable of walking in the Spirit. They do not forsake the gathering together of the saints in corporate worship and study, but can survive spiritually on their own if necessary. Truly, when we are born again, the "blood" of our spirit then changes from a basic form to that which can sustain spiritual life. He came that we might have life, and that life more abundant!

FEAST OF TABERNACLES
~ LUNG DEVELOPMENT

The LORD said to Moses, "Say to the Israelites; 'On the fifteenth day of the seventh month the LORD's Feast of Tabernacles begins, and it lasts for seven days. The first day is a sacred assembly; do no regular work. For seven days present offerings made to the LORD by fire, and on the eighth day hold a sacred assembly and present an offering made to the LORD by fire. It is the closing assembly; do no regular work. Leviticus 23:33-36

The tabernacle of the Lord was a tent constructed by Moses in the wilderness. The Spirit of God would dwell within the tabernacle, and Moses would go there for prayer and worship. The Holy Spirit is identified as a wind, as air, coming and going as He pleases. Christ breathed His Holy Spirit upon the disciples, showing us that He likens breath to the Spirit.

It is just as fascinating to realize that this feast, the feast of tabernacles that signified the Lord's dwelling within us through His Holy Spirit, is at the same time that the baby's lungs are developed enough to sustain life outside the womb, allowing them to sustain themselves with breath. A wonderful coincidence?

Growth In Christ:

Now that the Christian has grown in maturity, now that they have experienced the overflowing love for the Abba Father, they now cannot help but begin to use their breath to testify of the Lord. Their hearts begin to burn with an evangelical fire, as they desire to fulfill the Matthew 28:19 commission, to go out and make disciples of all nations.

When a person accepts Christ, they publicly declare their decision by being baptized in water. The disciples, even John the Baptist, did this with Jesus in their presence. However, Jesus said in Matthew 3:11, Mark 1:8, Luke 3:16, and John 1:33 that He, Himself, would baptize the new believer with the Spirit and fire. We see this happen to the disciples at Pentecost. Although they had been Christians, disciples of Christ, they weren't baptized with the Spirit until that day in the upper room after Jesus' ascension into Heaven.

It was then that they received the dunamis power (same word root used for the word dynamite) of the Holy Spirit, allowing them to receive spiritual gifts and manifestations. You have been saved by grace, and you are a Christian. Have you ever asked to receive this dunamis power of the Holy Spirit? Receiving the spiritual gifts and manifestations in an orderly way, according to scripture (1 Corinthians 12), is the most ultimate blessing the Christian can receive.

FEAST OF DEDICATION
~ BIRTH

"Then came the Feast of Dedication at Jerusalem. It was winter, and Jesus was in the temple area walking in Solomon's colonnade. The

Jews gathered around him, saying, 'How long will you keep us in
suspense? If you are the Christ, tell us plainly."
John 10:22 – 24

There was a ruthless Syrian leader in 165 BC, Antiochus Epiphanes, who was desecrating and destroying the Jewish Temple. Judah, the Maccabee, and his family formed a revolt against the Syrians. They miraculously defeated them and took back the Temple. In preparing to celebrate the victory, they were dismayed that the oil used to light the "candle of eternity," the Ner Hatamid, was nearly all discarded. Antiochus had polluted and destroyed most of their vessels of oil. The only acceptable vial of oil left was enough to last only one day.

God intervened on their behalf, however, and caused the oil to last an entire eight days and eight nights. This gave them time to prepare for more acceptable oil to keep the candle of eternity burning bright. Since then, the Jews have kept a Festival of Dedication of the Temple after regaining it back from Antiochus Epiphanes. This festival symbolizes a new beginning, and is celebrated today as Hanukkah.

Jesus, Himself, is seen in John, chapter four, celebrating Hanukkah. For us, it symbolizes not only the rebuilding and dedication of the temple, but also is the new feast added to the seven, completing this perfect picture of gestation. Hanukkah happens at 280 days after Passover, and those who have worked in the pregnancy field will recognize that number. It is the average length of pregnancy!

The picture is perfect, because as Hanukkah is a picture of a new beginning, so is the birth of a child an actual event that starts life outside the womb - a very new beginning for the little baby who was tucked nicely inside the mother's womb. God, in His wisdom, has placed this feast at the right time after Passover, to complete the gestational period of intrauterine growth. The eight days of the festival even allowed for the variables in the actual date of delivery from the due date. This is very fascinating, but even more intriguing is it's implications for salvation!

Growth In Christ:

The ultimate stage in the life of the Christian is the longing and the hope for Heaven. It is a mysterious thing to watch, as Christians who deeply love the Lord, worship Him in a way that exhibits a great desire to leave this world and spend eternity with the Lord in Heaven.

The sting of death is gone, and one's personal goal is to see the Lord return to gather His church from the four winds. What a glorious day that will be, when the dead in Christ will rise, our gestation here on Earth will be complete, and we will be born into the kingdom! Hallelujah and Amen!

There are many things in this world that point us to our Creator. The firmament, the predictability of an ocean wave, the torrent of a mighty wind, and the wonder of a tiny flower or insect all testify of His magnificent works. There are, however, very specific things that point not only to God the Creator, but to Jesus Christ, His Son.

Take, for example, Niagara Falls. Also referred to as "Horseshoe Falls," the carving of the cliff that creates the waterfall resembles the shape of an omega (Ω). How is this significant? Jesus said, "I am the Alpha and the Omega, the beginning and end." If Niagara Falls is in the shape of an omega, in order to see Christ etched into this beautiful landscape by the finger of God, there must somewhere be an Alpha representing a beginning.

Niagara Falls is well known as the "honeymoon capital of the world." How fitting, then, for the Lord to include His children in this beautiful depiction of Christ, with the representation of the alpha of love, beginning of life together, the marriage. What would the Lord be saying with this picture? I believe He would tell us that He is preparing a great marriage ceremony for us, His bride, the Church. He is the beginning of our love, for God is love. As the water cascades and falls into the river below, He desires for us to fall in love with Him, giving us a river of life flowing out of our innermost being.

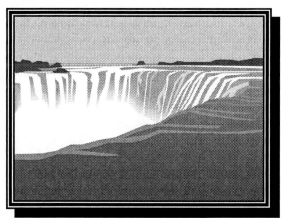

God wants us to be in love with Him, in love with Jesus Christ. He desires this so much, that he has not only placed His signature and approval of Jesus Christ on Niagara Falls, He has inscribed His plan for salvation into gestation of every pregnancy. He desires for us, as Christians, to grow and mature until that great day when we spend eternity with Him in Heaven.

Feast	Even in Pregnancy	Growth In Christ
Lamb Selection Day/ Palm Sunday	Pre-Conception	*"Before I formed you in the womb I knew you, before you were born I set you apart. Jeremiah 1:5*
Passover	Ovulation	Christ dies while the soon-to-be Christian is still "dead" in their transgressions
Unleavened Bread	Fertilization	Acceptance of Christ as personal Lord and Savior
First Fruits	Implantation	Acceptance of the all-sufficient nature of the blood of Christ and drawing near to the Lord.
Feast of Weeks (Pentecost)	Recognizably Human	Recognizable as a Christian by actions, by love
Feast of Trumpets	Hearing	Ability to hear the voice of God in the heart
Day of Blood Atonement	Hemoglobin A	Ability to take up the cross daily, and deny ourselves
Feast of Tabernacles	Lungs	Jesus baptizes with the Spirit and fire, and the Christian testifies through words, action, and love
Hanukkah	Birth	The Christian moves into the realm of eternal worship in the arms of their Lord! Hallelujah!

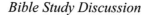

Bible Study Discussion

1. What is your reaction to the correlations between the feasts and pregnancy?

2. Share your knowledge and/or experience with the feasts. Perhaps there are still some unanswered questions...

3. What did you do to prepare your marriage for parenthood?

4. Where else can you see the signature of God in nature? For example, the crystals in the dried teardrop, when viewed under a microscope, form the shape of a cross. This could be the Lord reminding us that the Lord sees each tear we shed and is mindful of our pain. We ought to remember the cross in our tears, that He endured the ultimate pain, and understands and shares our pain.

5. Where are you in your pregnancy as it relates to the feasts?

Week of Pregnancy	Event of Pregnancy	
2	Pre-Conception	Lamb Selection
3 (Day one)	Ovulation	Passover
3 (Day two)	Fertilization	Unleavened Bread
4 (Day will vary)	Implantation	First Fruits
9/10	Recognizably a Fetus	Pentacost
28 + 0 days	Hearing is verified	Feast of Trumpets
29 + 3 days	Adult blood is formed	Day of Blood Atonement
30 + 1	Lungs are developed enough to survive life outside the womb	Feast of Tabernacles
(+/- 14 days)	Birth of baby	Hanukkah

Chapter Six
Fear Not

*For God hath not given us the spirit of fear; but of power,
and of love, and of a sound mind.*
2 Timothy 1:7

Parents, be on guard. Satan desires to sift you like wheat during pregnancy and delivery, and can easily do this with simple fear. Attacks of fear and doubt are often an hourly occurrence in the mind of expecting families, and can happen in the most unsuspecting places. It is difficult enough to battle the doubts that attack the mind, yet we also receive negative input from friends, family, and the media. Battling and overcoming fear is going to be your top priority, because the effects of fear and tension on pregnancy, labor, and delivery are often devastating.

Our bodies are made of three intertwined parts, the body, mind, and spirit. When one is under stress, it affects all three. Therefore, when the mind is under siege, the body interprets this as an unsafe environment for the baby to be born in and reacts by going into protective mode.

The meditations of the mind largely affect the womb, and eventually the baby. Fear, doubt, emotional stress, and tension all have negative effects on the process of birth, by directly affecting the uterus itself. It is important for you to know and understand the physiology of this phenomenon so that you can actively work to overcome it. In order to be successful, you will need to attack fear by controlling your body, the thoughts that you entertain in your mind, and most importantly your spirit.

The Physiology of Fear

Considered the pioneer of natural childbirth, Grantly Dick-Read, M.D. went against the medical model of childbirth during his day and presented to the world the radical idea that women could give birth normally and without excruciating pain. Dr. Read, having been a Christian himself, had stumbled upon a most wonderful discovery of human reproductive physiology that has been largely lost in today's information superhighway. Although much of his philosophy has been forgotten and replaced by modern pharmacology, many women are still blessed by his work. His book *"Childbirth Without Fear"* is a sought after work of art, and the truth in his discoveries is as timeless as ever and useful to us all. Dr. Read has wonderfully uncovered the mechanism used by the enemy to wreak havoc on the minds and bodies of laboring women. This section will detail his findings, explain how they work, and how you can apply them to your labor.

The Myometrium

The uterus is made up of three muscle layers called the *Myometrium*. Each layer has a separate function during birth, yet each are intertwined and become one large muscle.

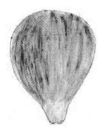 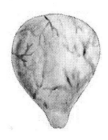 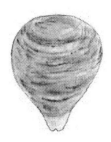

Outer Layer   **Middle Layer**   **Inner Layer**

The **outer layer** of the Myometrium has fibers that are laid out in a vertical pattern. These fibers are similar to those that you see in a piece of red meat at the supermarket, laid out in one direction forming a distinct visible pattern. The fibers of the outer layer start at the cervix, run up over the top of the uterus and down the back until they reach the cervix again. *It is this part of the uterus that is responsible for opening the cervix and pushing the baby out.*

The **middle layer** of the Myometrium is rich with blood vessels that supply the uterus and baby with nutrients and oxygen. The muscle fibers of the middle layer are arranged in a figure-eight pattern around each artery and vein. *The purpose of this layer is to support the blood vessels of the uterus.*

The **inner layer** of the Myometrium has fibers that are laid out in a horizontal pattern that encircle the uterus. Most of the fibers are close to the cervix and spread out until there are very few at the top. *The main function of this layer is to close the cervix and to shrink the uterus back down after the baby is born. The secondary function of this layer is to become rigid in an effort to <u>stall labor</u> if the mother has become fearful.*

When a woman is experiencing fear, she begins to resist the contractions by tensing up her body. By doing this, she triggers the *sympathetic nervous system,* which causes the inner layer of the uterus to resist dilation. Think back to a time when you were startled by something. What happened to your heart? It started beating faster, didn't it? Your heart began beating faster because there was an external stimulus that affected you mind, which triggered the sympathetic nervous system. Then your brain responded by dumping out adrenaline into your blood stream, which caused your heart to beat faster. The purpose of this was to prepare you to protect yourself or to run.

In just the same way, your uterus is affected by the sympathetic nervous system. The brain reacts to external stimuli (tension and/or fear) that can cause the inner muscle layer of the uterus to become rigid and resist the dilation efforts of the outer layer. As these two muscle layers work against each other, the uterus begins to feel stressed and *real clinical pain* develops.

Imagine yourself flexing your biceps. When your biceps are flexed, the opposing muscle (triceps) is relaxed, and vice versa. What would happen if another person were to try to straighten out your arm as you continued flexing? It would only take a few moments for your arm to begin to hurt, right?

When the inner muscle layer of the uterus becomes rigid, it puts resistance on the outer layer that is trying to dilate the cervix. Essentially, both opposing muscles are flexed at the same time, which induces a type of pain during childbirth that is unnatural. As you begin to feel this pain, you understandably become more tense and afraid. This *increases* the resistance of the inner layer and thus, a vicious cycle develops.

Activity to Try

Ask your husband to help you with this activity. Make a muscle for him with your biceps, and hold it there real tight. Ask him to try and straighten your arm out, while you resist his efforts. Have him time on his watch how long it takes for your muscle to become fatigued and begin to hurt.

Perhaps you are the athletic type, and you can last a good two to three minutes of resistance from your husband. That is great if you are only going to have a two-minute labor! After time, any woman would get fatigued from the resistance of the inner muscle trying to stall the birth due to fear.

Now repeat this exercise with the other arm, without the resistance of your husband. Make a muscle and hold it for 45 – 60 seconds at a time.

How did that feel? Not so bad, eh? It may have felt like a tension, but not necessarily painful. Finally, do it one more time, but this time, relax the rest of your muscles in your body including your face, take slow deep breaths, and place your mind into a tranquil state of rest. Repeat the flex for 60 seconds, rest for four minutes, and repeat the flex again. You will begin to see that a contraction, when not resisted, is really not all that bad.

Not only can pain be increased by tension and fear, the length of labor is greatly increased as well. As a matter of fact, some women are so frightened that they can get "stuck" at 3-4 centimeters and have to have a cesarean section due to dystocia (failure to progress). While all this is happening, the two muscles opposing each other pinch the blood vessels in the middle layer. Oxygen to the baby and uterus is reduced and serious complications can result.

Women are understandably afraid to go through labor and delivery. When a person is afraid of something, they tend to resist it by becoming tense. This inability to relax during labor is normal, yet can result with the inner layer of the uterus becoming rigid, creating much more pain than they would have normally experienced, as well as a lengthy labor; exactly what they were afraid of in the first place!

A Certified Nurse Midwife in Iowa had this experience:

This was a lady on her 4th baby. I asked the nurse to listen to heart tones while I did a check. Her cervix was 8 cm, 100% effaced, and that very soft, melt-away consistency where it would stretch open as wide as my fingers could spread. Just then, we heard a big dip in the heart rate. Immediately I felt the cervix close up to 6 cm or less, and a rigid half-centimeter thick. I believe this was due to the drop in baby's heart rate frightening the mom. Heart tones recovered, mom was reassured, and she was complete in another 10 minutes. ... I am a definite believer in the effect that fear has on the cervix during labor. Bernice Keutzer, CNM

It is important to remember that there are three potential outcomes of labor. The first possibility is what will happen if we are completely relaxed and without anxiety. This is the labor that the Lord intended for us to have. The second course of labor is what we experience if we are unable to control the thoughts and meditations that we maintain while in labor.

If we are continuing to say, "I don't like this," or "Lord, please just take the pain away - make it stop," then we are resisting the process with negative thoughts and that will begin the fear-tension-pain cycle. This course of labor will be one that is much more difficult and potentially less enjoyable. The third is if we will be facing an unnatural childbirth, managed with synthetic hormones. This is different situation entirely, and will be discussed in subsequent chapters.

We cannot control many things while in labor, but we can control our muscles, our spirit, our breathing, and our mind. By taking each thought captive and making it obedient to Christ, full of peace and yielding to the process, we actually can affect our labor directly. Taking charge of our countenance is a critical component to a joyful experience.

Quiet Thought

1. Do you believe that fear of pain can be overcome?

2. Who is adding to your fear, and who is helping reduce it?

3. What Bible story or scripture might correlate to the issue of overcoming fear?

4. How does Jesus Christ give us a peace that is not of this world?

5. Do you have faith that the Lord will deliver you from all your fears?

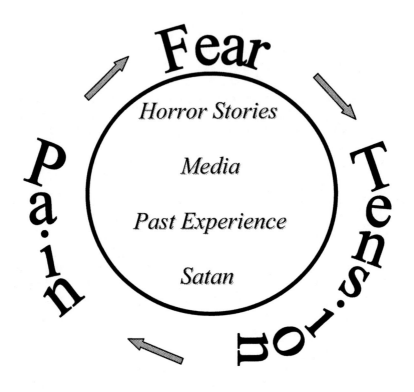

Fear

Tension

Pain

Horror Stories

Media

Past Experience

Satan

Prayer   Breathing

Scripture   Relaxation

Support Partner

Overcoming Fear

Most of us have a picture in our mind of a laboring woman who is writhing in pain, shouting obscenities, pulling hair, and crying out during the throws of labor. These women may never have been told about the principle of fear being one of the major causes of excruciating pain. Therefore, make every effort to maintain a sense of confidence, tranquility, safety, and control during contractions.

Regardless of what stage of labor you are in, it is critical for you to focus on four things. For the Christian, these four items conveniently work out into the perfect acronym – C.A.L.M. The acronym itself is a summation of all that we are to be during labor, no matter what is put on our plate. The c.a.l.m. acronym works out this way:

C - Christ Appropriately placed at the beginning, we need Christ above all else. Jesus promised us His Holy Spirit, who comforts us during labor. There is no room for the fear if we allow the peace of Jesus Christ to take over our entire being. How exactly do we access Christ during labor? Jesus said that wherever two or more are gathered, then He would be within their midst. You and your support partners can join in worship, prayer, communion, and meditation throughout your labor, all the while knowing that Jesus promised that He would be there. Jesus Christ, the Comforter and the One who takes away our fear, is the most powerful pain relief method that we could ever be given. Do not leave Him out!

A - Attitude The type of thoughts that are entertained in our minds during labor are extremely critical. They can literally alter the course of labor, changing the pain from bearable to abnormally acute. Rather than saying, "I can't do this. Don't make me do this," say "I've made it this far. I am going to focus on this contraction only, complete it, and focus on the here and now, rather than the road ahead of me. What I am doing right now is bringing me one contraction closer to my baby." No bad thoughts, just good, prayerful thoughts!

In addition to the thoughts that are entertained, it is equally important for you to achieve a state of mind that is drifting in and out of stage-one sleep. A mind that is in a lower state of consciousness is not fully aware of the work of the uterus, whereas a fully alert mind is keenly aware of every sensation. As labor intensifies, the mind should become increasingly dreamy and deep in relaxation. It is therefore beneficial to enter into a state of prayerful meditation that induces a sleep-like state of mind to lessen pain perception and aid in your ability to cope with the discomfort of labor.

L - Lungs Surprisingly, your breathing has a direct effect to how much pain you will experience. Slow, deep abdominal breathing is very effective in inducing a sleep-like state, helping the body to enter into deep relaxation. As mentioned before, if a person wants to slow down their racing heart, they take slow and deep breaths to counteract the sympathetic nervous system. This method is also useful for relaxing the inner muscle layer of the uterus, allowing the outer layer to do its work quicker and with less pain. Since abdominal breathing is the same type of breathing we use while sleeping, it is the perfect tool for helping us achieve the level of relaxation needed for coping with contractions.

M - Muscles The most difficult component of this acronym may very well be the ability to keep tension out of our muscles during a contraction. The automatic response to a building contraction is resistance. Our brows furrow, hands clench, elbows lock, backs arch, shoulders raise, and bottoms tighten in an attempt to fight against the pain. Letting every muscle loosen at the onset of a contraction takes practice, discipline, and determination. The reward of a less painful labor, however, is well worth the effort. Remember, one tense muscle can communicate to your body that there is a dangerous environment for the baby to be born into, creating a longer and more painful labor.

There are several recent studies in two new fields of study called psychosomatic and psychosocial obstetrics. They are very interesting and support the findings of Dr. Grantly Dick-Read, who asserted that anxiety during childbirth led to complications and a lower satisfaction with the birth experience. It is not a surprise that science is supporting the Biblical truth, which teaches us that fear is not of the Lord.

There is no fear in love, but perfect love
casts out all fear because fear has to do with torment.
1 John 4:18

The only one who has perfect fear is God Himself, and He is the one who can cast out our fear. We can give Him the responsibility, and not to worry about our ability to overcome it. In faith, we tell the Lord that we are counting on Him to take away fear from us. Tell Him that you believe in the scripture, and that His scripture said He would cast out all our fears, and He will.

We do have some responsibility in the matter, however. We can develop a short prayer paragraph, and greet each contraction with it when they come. Even if you are all alone, Jesus is the best birth coach there could ever be. He is our Comforter, and will indeed be there to comfort you.

Any negative thoughts are not from God, we know that. When you get a negative thought, just remind the author of that thought that you are saved, and that is all that really matters, so nothing that happens here on earth can take your eternity away from you. Remind him that Jesus suffered so much on the cross, for the JOY set before him, and you are prepared to join in that fellowship of suffering, that light affliction that lasts only a moment in time, for the joy of your child, the joy of the Father's child who is making their entrance to the world.

Things are so different when you approach labor with a peaceful mind; it is worth more than precious jewels. Even if you have the most painful and complicated birth that was ever recorded in history, you can go in and accomplish it with joy - counting yourself worthy of sharing in the sufferings of Christ. Every time you experience pain in the delivery room, rejoice like the apostles, who were excited to have been able to experience a fraction of what their Lord experienced. Greet each contraction, welcome it with prayer, and give it permission to accomplish its task.

You have a huge amount of control over what goes on in your mind. When it comes to fear, you can trust in God that He will be the One to take it away. This great relief frees you to meditate on things that are true and beautiful. Turn negative thoughts into prayers for others. Pray for your baby's salvation. After the next negative thought, pray for your baby's future spouse's salvation. Teach Satan that each time he attacks you with a negative and fearful thought; it will generate prayer of salvation for someone else. Pray over your birth, how you want it to go - perfectly, just as God's perfect will is. If He wants you to join Christ in suffering, then so be it. Rejoice in that. If he wants you to have an easy two-hour birth, then that's okay too. Get excited about what God is going to do, what His good and perfect will is, and pray that you want only that and nothing else.

The Control Factor

In a low-risk pregnancy, when everything is normal, there is a multitude of decisions that will affect your labor and delivery. Sometimes one of the biggest issues to overcome is surrendering control of the birth process. How much should we let go of? To what extent should we allow others to care for us as we journey into labor? Indeed, there are aspects of the birth that should be surrendered, yet there are things that you will need to manage yourself. It is not wise to put each and every decision into the hands of your care provider. They do expect that you will be doing research about birth management and they should offer you to articulate those choices by means of a birth plan.

If the birth plan is neglected, the door to disappointment may be opened and you may find yourself regretting certain aspects of the experience. If, however, you have done all of your homework and learned as much as you can about procedures, and something does happen that you didn't want or the birth plan isn't realized, you at least know that you gave it your best effort in preparing.

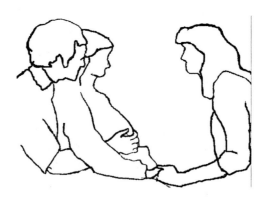

Column A

Things You CAN control in a normal labor	Comments	Considerations
Location of Birth	Wherever you birth, it should be where YOU feel most safe. This will ensure that you are able to relax and let your body deliver the baby.	Make sure that they are willing to honor your birth plan, and have a reputation of doing so.
Your choice of provider	Do your own research. Don't choose a provider because that is where your friend went. Rather, interview them, speak with past patients, ask to see their statistics for cesarean vs. natural births, etc.	This is critical. If you are not comfortable, you have the right to change your provider at any time. YOU employ them, not the other way around. Go with who you feel will take the time to listen to you and honor your wishes the best.
Who will be your birth team	Chose who will be of most comfort and help to you.	Many will want to be with you, and it is important that you choose carefully who can be there. Will they be a spectator only, or will they actually help you?
What interventions you will allow	If your labor is normal, there is no reason for any intervention. Labor is best when left undisturbed.	It is difficult to deliver a true informed consent during labor regarding procedures. It is up to you to study before hand to know the true risks and benefits.
Your position for labor and for birth	There are many beneficial positions for labor and delivery, and you can take advantage of more of them when you are not hindered by many unnecessary procedures.	Unless you have approved of certain procedures, which limit your movement. Example: IV prevents shower/jacuzzi, external monitor prevents active walking, and an epidural prevents any movement from the waist down.

Column B

Things You Cannot Control	Your State of Mind	Scripture
When labor will begin	Pray for perseverance during the uncomfortable stages. Provided everything is fine with you and baby, it is incredibly important to let labor begin naturally. Isaiah 40:31	*Isaiah 40:31* *Psalm 130* (Entire Psalm)
Who will be delivering your baby (if you are with a group of provides)	Remember that the provider often times is not present for the vast majority of the labor. Those present with you for the first stage of labor are the most important to you. (Another great reason to have a doula)	*Psalm 139:7-10*
How long labor will last	Let go of the need to know how long it will take. Take one contraction at a time, not worrying how long it has taken or how long you have to go. Say, "Now that is one contraction closer to my baby." In the throws of labor, begin to focus on one breath at a time. Be in the moment, focus on your breathing, which _is_ controlled. This will indirectly control the length of your labor. Paradoxically, by letting go of control, you can control it.	*Leviticus 23:4* The feasts had their appointed time, and contractions have their appointed time. Receive each one with joy, knowing it is the source of what brings your child.
The baby will come out.	Release fears about the baby passing through the birth canal. Any thought about the pain, chance of tear, or sexuality of it should be cast out. Let your mind work with your body to open and permit the baby to come down.	*Psalm 71:6*

If you are unable to overcome fear and/or tension, then unnatural pain and perhaps other complications begin to be added to the situation. Labor is no longer taking the normal course of events, but rather one that may include unnecessary discomfort or procedures. You are in control of many things during labor, but the single most important thing you should be concerned with is the state of your mind. If you are able to control this with prayerful thoughts and meditations, then you have a great effect on the events of labor.

It might seem like there are many things that you cannot control during birth, but in reality, many of those things will be affected by your mind. The length of labor, the intensity of labor, and the health of the baby could very well have an indirect link to the confidence and serenity of the mother. Again, while many issues in birth are unavoidable, what can be taken charge of is the activity of your mind.

We demolish arguments and every pretension that sets itself up
against the knowledge of God, and we take captive
every thought to make it obedient to Christ.
2 Corinthians 10:5

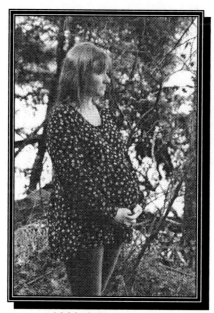

1998 © Townsend

Bible Study Discussion

1. How have you begun to prepare for the birth of your child?

2. Do you struggle with any fears about birth?

3. Discuss the fear-tension-pain process and how you plan to avoid it.

4. Where do you want to maintain control over the process and where do you plan to surrender control?

5. What part of this chapter stands out to you?

Chapter Seven
Armor of God

The birth of a family, or new family member, is a sacred event. The enemy would desire it to become a spiritual battleground, hoping to infiltrate it in subtle ways that can cause frustration and guilt, in order to compromise the family's foundations. Satan knows that if he can scramble the peace and confidence in the parent's mind, then he has a good foothold from the start. As parents, it is good to be prepared for this attack in advance, praying for a hedge of protection around you.

The Bible tells us that we can stand during these attacks by putting on the spiritual armor of God. We can stand therefore, literally and figuratively, as we take authority over our minds by putting on the articles of defense God has given us.

Ephesians 6:10-13
[10]Finally, be strong in the Lord and in his mighty power. [11]Put on the full armor of God so that you can take your stand against the devil's schemes. [12]For our struggle is not against flesh and blood, but against the rulers, against the authorities, against the powers of this dark world and against the spiritual forces of evil in the heavenly realms. [13]Therefore put on the full armor of God, so that when the day of evil comes, you may be able to stand your ground, and after you have done everything, to stand.

Paul begins this passage with "Finally," and uses it as if he is saving the best for last; the most important point of all. He reminds us to be strong, as a friend would encourage another to be strong in a tough situation. It suggests that there will be trials coming our way, things that are going to happen that we will need to be protected from. Jesus reminded us that we WILL have trials and tribulations in this world, but "Behold, I have overcome the world," He said.

It is important to keep in mind that the battle was fought and the victory has already been established when Jesus said "It is finished" on the cross. Satan lost that day, and we now know that our salvation is secure in Christ Jesus, as we wait for His return. Satan only has victory when we *give in* to Him. With that said, the rest of this passage gives us tools to help us from not giving into the lies of the enemy.

Put on the full armor of God so that you can take your stand against the devil's schemes. Ephesians 6:11

Satan works against us by using schemes, plans, and other ways that will separate us from the Lord. He is like a woodpecker searching for a bug on a tree. The woodpecker does not hammer away at the tough area of bark, but rather he pecks away until he finds a weak area and then drills it, because he knows there is a bug underneath. So too, Satan does not waste time on our strong points, but finds our weaknesses because he wants to devour us.

Blessed is the man who perseveres under trial, because when he has stood the test, he will receive the crown of life that God has promised to those who love him.
James 1:12

For our struggle is not against flesh and blood, but against the rulers, against the authorities, against the powers of this dark world and against the spiritual forces of evil in the heavenly realms.
Ephesians 6:12

How hard it is to remember this verse when someone else has hurt us! Keep a watchful eye out for Satan, who stands behind the hurtful person, and gives a quiet sinister laugh. May we begin to pray for the person Satan has used, and lift them before the Lord. May we monitor our own life, making sure that we don't have a devil behind us, laughing because we have just been used to hurt someone else.

Therefore put on the full armor of God, so that when the day of evil comes, you may be able to stand your ground, and after you have done everything, to stand. Ephesians 6:13

Of course the day of labor and delivery is hardly evil, but Satan would like to make it that way. It doesn't have to be, and no matter what happens, you can have perfect peace in your mind and in your heart, knowing that God is going to bless you and your family with an abundance of love. As you put on your armor, proclaim that your day is covered in God's grace and that you will not allow Satan into this experience. Resist him, and he must flee!

Belt of Truth

Stand firm then, with the belt of truth buckled around your waist…
Ephesians 6:14

The cloth belt was used to gather up the lengthy garment so that the warrior could run without tripping, giving him freedom of movement. The act of gathering up the garment, or "girding one's self," can be likened to preparing the mind with the truth and facts about childbirth. If you understand what each and every intervention's implications have on the birth, then you are well prepared to run and move about in the battle for normalcy in childbirth.

"We have learned all that we can about the pros and cons of all the decisions that we have to make. We ask for your perfect will, Lord. Help us to be discerning and wise in these areas, and Holy Spirit, impart truth in all areas of this birth."

Breastplate of Righteousness

…with the breastplate of righteousness in place…
Ephesians 6:14

Integrity and honorable behavior bring a shining light to a dark world. Conversely, when we engage in behavior that is unholy, we remove the breastplate from our spiritual self. Without this article of armor, the vital organs are left exposed to injury. The heart is vulnerable to becoming wounded or hardened.

"We will not act in a way that is unbecoming or rude. We will be a great witness for our Lord, Jesus Christ. Bring others to us, Lord, that will need to see you through us. Help us to have a gentle and quiet spirit, yet firm and confident in birth.

Shoes of Readiness

...and with your feet fitted with the readiness that comes from the gospel of peace. Ephesians 6:15

Much like the belt of truth, this article of armor was to allow for free movement without pain on the feet. We need to be prepared to move out quickly in many circumstances, and if we have readied ourselves, it will be far less painful than being unprotected.

"I will do all that I can to prepare my body, my soul, and my spirit. I will equip myself with scripture, prayer, and self-control. I will be ready to testify to my beliefs about my Lord, Jesus Christ to anyone who inquires of me. I will preach the gospel by my actions, and if necessary, use words."

Shield of Faith

In addition to all this, take up the shield of faith, with which you can extinguish all the flaming arrows of the evil one.
Ephesians 6:16

The most important thing to remember about faith is that it is not an emotion. Exercising faith is when we know that God's promises will be kept, regardless of the circumstances. In our frailty, we are prone to worry and doubt, but as we learn to rely on God for our every need, we begin to witness His power, and it is not so difficult then to trust that He will remove our fears and doubts when the time comes. Even when we are faithless, He remains faithful and we can invest in that truth so that when we waiver, we know we have Him to fall back on. Once this faith is established, all the horror stories in the world couldn't move us into a place of worry and doubt, because we have our Redeemer!

"We believe in the promise of the Comforter, that is given to those who live by faith. We believe that the Holy Spirit can comfort us during this time, and we put our hope in Him, to allow us to have a beautiful birth experience that He desires us to have. We will not allow the fiery darts of Satan to put fear into our minds. We have the faith that God's perfect love can cast out any fear that comes our way. We do not put our faith

in man, but in the Creator of man. Our faith in our providers is limited to the loving grace that you have shed on us all. We ask for you to give our providers wisdom, Lord, guide and direct their hands. We believe that You will calm our hearts by the oil of the Holy Spirit."

Helmet of Salvation

Take the helmet of salvation…
Ephesians 6:17

The Holy Spirit will guide us in all situations, writing the Lord's will upon the tablets of our heart, giving us heavenly wisdom, discernment, diplomacy, judgment, and understanding, that we can draw upon under any circumstance.

We enjoy all of these things because we have the knowledge of our secure salvation in Christ, which protects our minds from fear and worry about pain, adequate care, and even death. We can go therefore, being confident that He will direct our paths.

Sword of the Spirit

…and the sword of the Spirit, which is the word of God.
Ephesians 6:17

Possibly the most effective tool against fear is faith. The Bible says that faith comes by hearing, and hearing by the Word of God. Daily scripture reading has a unique quality to it that allows the Lord to speak to us intimately. As we study through a book in the Bible, the chapter we are reading for that day often times will speak directly to the situation that we are dealing with at that time. The more this happens, the more we trust that the Bible is a living document, almost breathing with life, as seen in Hebrews 4:12. When we begin to trust in the power of the Holy Spirit within the pages of the Bible, we begin to trust in the promises written there regarding the Lord's ability to take away our fear and to keep us safe in His arms.

"We have hidden Your word in our heart, that we might not sin against You, Lord. Also, we have brought along many scriptures to help us during the birth of our child."

Prayer In The Spirit

And pray in the Spirit on all occasions with all kinds of prayers and requests. With this in mind, be alert and always keep on praying for all the saints.
Ephesians 6:18

"Lord, we ask you to help us to be in the Spirit at all times, as we pray without ceasing. Lord, may our lives be lived as a prayer to you. We will meditate on your Word, and believe the promises that you have given us, speaking them back to you. God, help us to keep our eyes fixed on you as your child is born. Thank you for giving us this baby, and help us to train him or her up in Your ways so that they may not depart from it when they are older. Thank you, in Jesus' name, Amen!

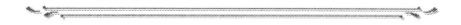

Bible Study Discussion

1. Has there been any spiritual warfare during this pregnancy?

2. How are you combating these issues?

3. How have others been an encouragement to you, or a hindrance?

4. How is your walk with the Lord?

5. How have you gone on the offense in the spiritual battle of today?

Chapter Eight
The Basics of Birth

One way fear can build up in our mind is through the unknown. A brief overview of the female reproductive system and the process of birth will help you to understand the basic course of events that you can expect while you are delivering your baby. It is not necessary to delve into a complete physiological graduate study on the process of birth, but it is wise to familiarize yourself so there might not be any surprises.

Anatomy

Uterus – The uterus (womb) is where the baby spends the entire nine months of pregnancy. Before pregnant, it is the size and shape of a small upside down pear. As the baby grows, the uterus stretches and enlarges respectively. An interesting feature that the Lord built into pregnancy is that the measurement of the uterus from the pubic bone to the fundus (top part of the uterus) generally corresponds with how many weeks pregnant you are. For example, if you are 24 weeks pregnant, then more than likely your fundus will be 24 cm above the top edge of your pubic bone.

Placenta – The placenta is a temporary organ that develops out of the amniotic sac and usually attaches itself to the upper back wall of the uterus. It acts as an exchange organ that filters out *some* toxins from the mother's blood, passes oxygen and nutrients to the baby, and allows for waste to be returned to the mother's blood stream. Although the mother's and baby's blood never mixes, much of the contents is shared via osmosis. After the delivery of the baby, the placenta detaches itself from the uterus and is passed outside the body, causing pregnancy to completely end.

Umbilical Cord – Attached from the placenta to the abdomen of the child, the umbilical cord is the lifeline to the mother's nurturing. The umbilical cord has two arteries carrying waste products from the baby to the mother, and one vein carrying nutrients from the mother to the baby. This cord will be severed after the baby is born, leaving a short stub on the baby's tummy that will eventually fall off. What is left is the navel or bellybutton. This will be severed at birth, leaving a short stub, and will eventually fall off and what is left is the navel.

Amniotic Sac and Fluid – This is what is commonly referred to as the "bag of waters," where the baby will float around in for the entire pregnancy. The fluid acts as a cushioning device for the baby, keeps the baby at a constant temperature, allows for movement and exercise, and provides some nutrients as the baby drinks the fluid throughout pregnancy. The amniotic fluid has been estimated to be exchanged at a rate of about 500 ml per hour, being completely exchanged about every three hours.

Cervix - This may be one of the most miraculous events of labor and delivery. This small muscular opening at the bottom of the uterus will go from completely closed to opening to a full four inches, or what is more commonly referred to as 10 centimeters. Not only does the cervix open to this diameter, it also thins out until it essentially disappears up the side of the uterus until medical personnel can no longer detect it. This process of first stage labor is called dilation (opening of the cervix) and effacement (thinning out of the cervix).

Effacement

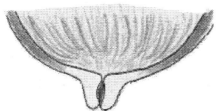

0% Effaced (Both openings of the cervix are closed)

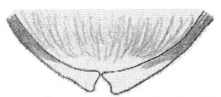

50% Effaced Bottom part of cervix is dilating, but the inner opening is still closed

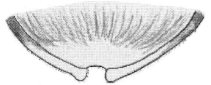

75% Effaced Cervix is almost 2 cm

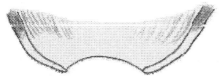

90% Effaced Cervix is about 6 cm

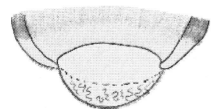

100% Effaced Cervix cannot be felt by medical personnel.

The Basic Process of Birth

You will notice that in order for the baby to come out of the body, she must first pass through the cervix and the vagina. In order for this to happen, the cervix will need to open large enough for the baby to exit into the vagina. This process is called the "first stage" of labor. The second stage of labor is after the cervix completely dilates and the baby begins to enter the birth canal. Birth happens when the body of the baby is completely out of the mother's birth canal, however the umbilical cord and placenta are still within the confinements of the uterus. The attendant will cut the umbilical cord and hand you the baby while they wait for the placenta to be delivered, which is the third and final stage of labor.

False Labor

How can you be sure that you are really in labor? Most of us know of someone who rushed off to the hospital only to be turned away due to a "false alarm." It is comforting to know that these early contractions are really the uterus exercising itself in preparation for the birth. Not necessarily false labor, these "Braxton-Hicks" contractions are useful and serve an important purpose – to strengthen and ready the uterus for the event of birthing your child.

Braxton Hicks Contractions – The uterus is exercising for labor, and becomes rigid and hard. The contractions may be very rhythmical and constant, or irregular and unpredictable, but do not increase in their intensity, nor do they make significant changes to the cervix. Drinking a tall glass of water or changing positions may alleviate the contractions. Not every woman has Braxton-Hicks contractions, however, the more the uterus can exercise, the stronger it will be for labor. Stimulation of the uterus can cause these contractions, so remaining active in late pregnancy seems to go hand in hand with a stronger uterus. Stronger uterus = faster labor! Check with your care provider to make sure mild activity is okay. Also, if you are less than 37 weeks and you begin to have rhythmical contractions or a low dull ache that radiates around to your back, that do not go away after drinking plenty of water and changing your activity, you may want to inform your care provider to rule out whether labor has begun earlier than it should.

True Labor

Possible Signs

1. Loose Bowels – The body is preparing for labor by making more room in the pelvis. Loose bowels or even diarrhea with a flu-like feeling can occur prior to the onset of labor. Although not an absolute sign of labor, it is a good sign that the body is getting ready.
2. Nesting Instinct – One of the more exciting anecdotes told by ladies is the urge to prepare the home for the arrival of the baby. Not everyone gets it, but those who do tell that there was an unmistakable burst of energy in the hours preceding the onset of labor. Nesting is probably brought on by hormonal changes (prostaglandins) that are associated

with the softening of the cervix. Make sure not to overdo it during this time as you will need to conserve your energy for the birth!

3. Backache – A low, dull backache sometimes precedes the onset of labor. You might have the need to keep changing positions.
4. Cramping – Intermittent or continuous cramps that radiate into the thighs.

Preliminary Signs

Mucous Plug - When the cervix begins to change, the mucous that blocked the uterus from germs, slips out. It looks much like egg white and may be tinged with light pink to red blood. This is sometimes referred to as the bloody show, but many times there is no blood and it can be passed without notice. It is not a definite sign of labor because a lady can lose her plug days or weeks before labor begins. It is a sign, however, that the cervix is beginning to change! NOTE: After a vaginal exam or intercourse, it is normal to pass a little blood, and it is often brownish in color. Any blood that is bright red needs to be reported to the care provider.

5. Amniotic Fluid Leak – Not necessarily a sure sign that labor has begun because there can be a leak without the onset of contractions. Occurs before labor about 10 – 12 percent of the time. A leak will sometimes seal over.
6. Braxton Hicks contractions   - contractions that do not increase in frequency, strength, length. However, they can accomplish mild changes in the cervix in preparation for true labor.

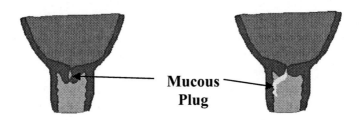

Mucous Plug

Positive Signs

7. Contractions That Create Cervical Change – contractions occur at regular and increasingly shorter intervals, and become longer and stronger in intensity.
8. Spontaneous Rupture of Membranes – this is usually followed by progressing contractions within a few hours. About 20% of all births begin this way.

The Phases of First Stage Labor

Phase One - Early Labor

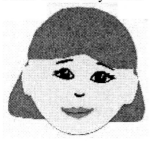

Early labor is from 0-3 centimeters, and can sometimes take many hours. Although it is the longest part of labor, it is generally the easiest. Most women will have a lifted countenance, and be able to talk through each contraction with ease.

If labor begins during the day, most women will try to go about their daily activities, trying not to become overly preoccupied with the contractions. Doing dishes, sweeping the floor, or organizing the baby's dresser are all things that moms do to keep busy during the early stages of labor. If she is in the hospital, she can be reading the Bible, slow dancing with her partner to worship music, walking through the halls, rocking in a rocking chair, going through the baby bag, etc. During the contraction, she eases her task, begins a cleansing abdominal breath, and says a gentle prayer to her Savior.

If labor begins at night, then she wakes for the contraction. Remaining in a confident and relaxed state, she gently takes slow abdominal breaths and prays, slipping back into sleep between the contractions. This will go on until she enters into active labor and needs to get up and more actively cope with her labor.

The Details of Early Labor

Contractions are timed from the *start of one contraction to the start of the next.* Early labor can have a sporadic pattern, where one contraction set is five minutes apart and another is longer. As labor progresses, a definite pattern should present itself, and the contractions will come on with greater predictability.

The actual length of the early labor contraction is generally 30 – 45 seconds, and mild in strength. This stage can last anywhere from 4 to 12 hours or more. If a woman is in writhing pain during early labor, it is *usually* because she has found herself in the middle of a fear-tension-pain cycle and her pain is abnormal. This can be turned around with helpful coaching, willingness on her part, and fervent prayer for C.A.L.M. If she is still experiencing acute pain, then her provider may need to make further assessments of the situation. For most women, however, early labor is a beautiful time between her and her husband as they enjoy their last few hours together before embarking on the journey to parenthood.

Phase Two - Active Labor

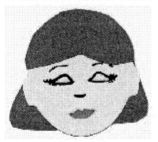

The countenance of a woman in active labor begins to change. No longer is she laughing at all the jokes or having conversations during the contractions, but now she is getting serious about the task at hand by using her concentration to remain calm and serene.

Between contractions, she is still able to interact with her attendants, but needs full attention to her work when the uterus acts. Family members may need to think about going to another room so that she can enter into a state of tranquility in the Lord. Many women want to entertain the friends and family, or don't want to hurt feelings if they ask them to leave. If the presence of a person is not aiding her in her ability to cope, then now is the time for them to go grab a nap or a bite to eat. After the cervix is completely dilated and she is focused on pushing, the family may be welcomed back in to witness the birth of their special little person.

Active labor is from 4 – 6 centimeters dilated, and usually lasts about 2 – 4 hours in length. Contractions last for about sixty seconds and are 3 – 7 minutes apart. It is the time that the decision to cope or escape is generally made.

Now is the time to ensure that you are in an upright position, if at all possible. It is tempting to get back into bed, but without the gravity of the baby's head pressing against the cervix, it will take longer to dilate. The weight of the baby against the cervix helps to thin it out and open it up. Think of it as sucking on that Lifesaver; the baby's head helps to melt it away. There's a new popular slogan that says, "Get up, and give birth!" There's truth in that.

The contractions of active labor have established a pattern, last longer, and come closer together. It is very important to seek the Lord in His help for your state of mind during this time. If you desire to get through childbirth without the use of interventions, it is important for you to know that this is the time when most women begin to experience self-doubt, and may give up and ask for relief. Determination, knowledge of the risks of every procedure, prayer, and remaining c.a.l.m. will help you to achieve your goal of natural childbirth.

Phase Three - Transition

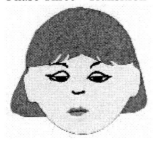

The countenance of women during transition takes on the form of total concentration and the deep need for sleep between contractions. The abdominal breaths become shallower and shorter, but still slow and under control. A loving coach can help you to breathe through the contractions, looking you square in the eyes and breathing with you.

Although this is the most intense part of labor, it is also the shortest. Every effort should be made to prevent the resistance of the body and mind to the process of transition. Your cervix will be opening from 7 to 10 centimeters in preparation for the baby to be born. You may begin to sweat, tremble, become nauseous, and/or weak under the great work of the uterus. All of these things are normal signs of progress and evidence that your body is working very hard. When they are seen, they can be celebrated because it only means that the baby should be coming soon!

If you give in to the temptation of resisting the efforts of the uterus now, you may be in for a difficult experience. It has happened far too often that a woman gets "stuck" at 8 centimeters and labors in transition for hours. This phase normally lasts 1 – 3 hours and no one would want to remain in a holding pattern with this level of discomfort. It is now that you will use all the strength that you own to remain calm and confident as your body completes the work that prepares the way of the baby. The power of transition can be frightening, but the power of the Lord to calm you is far greater and praise Him that he is able to do exceedingly more than we could ever expect!

The Details of Transition

If the contractions last 90 seconds, and they come every 2 minutes, that means that there is only 30 seconds between each contraction. Additionally, when the transition contraction begins to come down, it can have a "piggy-back" contraction that comes back up again. This is normal and is a sign that things are really moving along. Greet each one of the transition contractions with thanksgiving, knowing that they are bringing you one step closer to your baby.

Second Stage (Pushing)

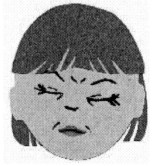

For most women, the incredible urge to bear down comes on very strong and is often irresistible. Now is the time to get into a good position and focus all of your efforts to your bottom. The pushing sensation of second stage labor is very similar to having a bowel movement. Because the little head is pushing on the nerves in the rectum, it mimics the feeling of going to the bathroom. Although intimidating, this is the feeling to go for while pushing, because these are the muscles needed to achieve the birth of the baby. This is very natural and should not be frightening to you. (For pushing techniques, see chapter seven.)

Details of Second Stage

The contractions of second stage labor are often far more manageable than the contractions needed to dilate the cervix, and many women report that it actually "feels good" to push. Provided that the baby is in a good position, the mom is not afraid of pushing, she can feel the sensations to push, and there are no abuse issues, this stage should progress nicely. There is more time between contractions to rest, and the intensity and sensations are largely different than anything she has experienced so far. The process of delivering the baby should take anywhere from one push to 3 hours, depending on how many children the mom has had and what position she is in.

Third Stage (Delivery of the Placenta)

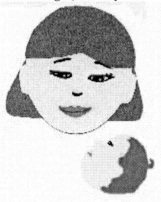

Praise the Lord, her baby's here! Now, for the first time, she will gaze into the eyes of her child and bond with kisses and squeals of delight. Things hoped for will now be realized and a new love relationship will ensue. This first hour of bonding is one that she will never forget, and should be sought after with great determination. There are very few instances when the baby should be taken for resuscitation,

116

but for the rest of the routine procedures, they can wait! If at all possible, the baby should remain with mother and father until the first feeding.

In the mean time, the placenta will be coming down the birth canal to be delivered. The contractions of the uterus "unzip" the placenta and after it is detached completely, it will gently be born into the attendant's basin. The baby nursing at the breast will cause uterine contractions that close off the blood vessels, preventing hemorrhage. God has designed the body to work just right to accomplish each task perfectly, and taking the baby away from mom interrupts His plan. Praise the Lord that He gave us the skilled attendants to help with the abnormal situations, but we also can praise Him that His design is perfect and can be trusted! Welcome little one!

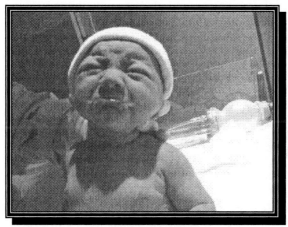

Copyright © Tripp 2004

Time To Practice

It is important to gain control over the processes of your body. From here on out, I want you to do this by letting go of every tension in your mind, your breath, and your muscles. When you get command of this, you will be more equipped to control your labor by letting go of all tension. Again, here are some activities to practice that of course are on a lesser level than a contraction, but will help you learn discipline over your body. They may sound trivial and a little humorous, but indeed they are effective.

1. When you develop an itch, purpose not to scratch it. This can be impossible at first, but with the control of the mind, abdominal breathing, and determination, you can learn to ride out the temptation to alleviate the discomfort. Marching band and military members must master this trick in order to not "break ranks," giving a sloppy appearance. By learning this technique, you will be able to reframe your perception of the sensations you are experiencing. Use the same technique to make it through a contraction without tensing up, diminishing pain.

2. Toileting practice. When you are going to have a bowel movement, practice accomplishing this without bearing down at all. See if you are able to allow your bowels to do all of the work by being totally relaxed. You will notice that it may take some sort of activity to get your mind off the bowel movement and on to something else like reading or counting. Once you occupy your mind with something other than the task at hand, you trick your mind into forgetting about the vulnerability of what you are doing and everything relaxes. Furthermore, your body might even give you a preview of what the involuntary urge to push is like. If you give your body total control over the bowel movement, it may induce a small-scale pushing reflex that is much like second-stage labor.

During birth, you are also vulnerable and your body instinctively will tense up. There are muscles there that you cannot control, but involuntarily tighten under times of stress. It takes distraction and relaxation of that area to allow them to let go and let "nature take its course." This is an example of how important it is to be confident through the vulnerability during birth, or the body will attempt to prevent the birthing of the baby. Use these exercises to learn how to work with, or in spite of, your body. The mind is powerful.

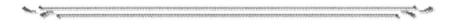

Bible Study Discussion

1. Watch a birth video that is positive and discuss it.

Order from www.cuttingedgepress.net

2. Do you understand the phases and stages of labor? What questions do you have?

3. What part of this chapter stands out to you?

4. What are your sources for learning inromation?

5. What decisions are you making, if any, based off of fear or emotion?

Chapter Nine
Practical Application For Labor

In this chapter, you will find techniques that may help during the first stage of labor. Keep in mind that there is no one way to give birth and these techniques are those that have helped women in the past, but may not be right for you during your labor.

I want to give permission to every woman to trust in her own God-given instinct to give birth normally and to know that the Lord will guide and direct you during this process. These techniques are here to help you gain understanding from women who have gone on before and have found these things to be helpful. I believe that we should "fill our bag" with as many ideas as possible so that when we do go into labor, we are well equipped. What may seem like a good idea before labor may not work during labor and whatever worked during early labor may not work during active labor. It is important to be as prepared and as flexible as possible. Although birth may not go as planned, even the most interventive birth can be Christ-centered and useful for glorifying God.

The Details

1. Breathing - There's no trick to it, no special pattern to memorize. No he he, haw haw's, just deep cleansing breaths from the diaphragm. Okay, take two deep breaths. Did your chest and shoulders rise? If so, you are breathing from the rib cage. *Rib cage breathing* uses the muscles between each rib, called the intercostals muscles, to draw air into your lungs by expanding the rib cage. *Abdominal breathing*, on the other hand, uses the diaphragm to expand the lungs. Now, take two more breaths, but this time keep your shoulders down and extend your abdomen. You will know that you are doing it correctly by placing your hand on your belly when you breathe in. If your hand is moving in and out with your belly as you breathe, you're doing it correctly. By taking slow abdominal breaths, (in through the nose, out through the mouth) you are filling your lungs up with the maximum amount of oxygen possible.

Imagine that your chest and abdomen are one of those ice-cream push up pops. You push up the plunger, and the ice cream goes up. You pull the plunger, and the ice cream goes down. Much like the plunger, the diaphragm goes up and down drawing air in and pushing it out. When you breathe in, it is as if you are pulling down the plunger drawing air into your lungs. As the diaphragm pushes downward, the abdominal organs are pushed outward, thus, making your stomach go out.

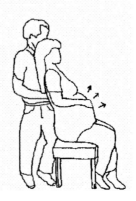

During labor, have your partner watch your breathing patterns and help you to remember to breathe from your diaphragm. Sometimes I have seen partners tell the mom "breathe, honey" over and over again. A stern "I AM breathing, darn it," usually follows! Sitting in front of you, and breathing with you, is often the best way your partner can encourage you to continue on. Some helpful words are "stay on top of it, don't resist it, that's the way, good," and so on.

In the original church, Christ breathed on the apostles and they received the Holy Spirit. I like to suggest that you try saying to yourself when you breathe in that you are breathing in the comfort of the Holy Spirit, and exhaling tension.

Some methods teach abdominal breathing combined with tapping into an internal strength to overcome fear and pain during birth. You will find with the Christ-centered childbirth approach, however, that the practice of going within yourself to find relaxation and pain relief is not so important, but that of bringing the Holy Spirit within yourself and leaning on Him for your comfort. Big difference!

Practice

Early & Active Labor

- Get into a comfortable position
- Rest your hands on your stomach
- Take a slow deep breath in for the count of four, making your hands rise (You only need to put hands on your abdomen until abdominal breathing comes natural to you and you get the hang of it – it is not necessary to do during labor)
- Hold your breath for the count of two
- Feel the tension and toxins releasing from your lungs and into your exhalation breath
- Very slowly, breathe out for the count of eight to ten
- Hold for one to two counts

Every time you breathe in say, "In with the Lord."
Every time you breathe out say, "Out with the tension" or "Out with the enemy."

Transition

- Breath in for the count of two to three
- Hold long enough to grab any tension and let it go
- Exhale for the count of four
- Hold for one count before repeating

The idea is to breathe a little slower than you naturally want to breathe. Women in transition tend to breath quite rapidly and can hyperventilate. Most will not be able to do deep abdominal breathing at this time, but slower controlled breathing is helpful in remaining calm and relaxed during a potentially intense time.

2. Body control - As stated before, even a clenched fist can stimulate the nervous system response that slows labor. It is ***critically important*** to be mindful of your body position throughout labor. Have your birth partners keep a constant watch for signs of tension in your face, hands, shoulders, back, jaw, and even your bottom. The goal is to try and keep as many muscles relaxed as possible during a contraction.

This does not mean lie in bed the entire time, however tempting that may be. As a matter of fact, most women find it extremely uncomfortable lying in bed during hard labor and do better by getting up. Try to remain upright as much as possible. This will help put pressure on the cervix, which facilitates dilation and effacement and speeds labor. As you are laboring upright, find a way to use only the muscles needed to keep you supported. If you are leaning into your partner, for instance, let them support you with their arms so that you can drop your own arms down, keeping them loose.

3. Mind Control - For most women, there are times in labor that can be mentally overwhelming. I have often seen women at five centimeters break down and give up, thinking that they have an equal amount of time to go from 5 to 10 cm as it took to get from 0 to 5cm. They feel that if this is how it feels to them at five centimeters, how can they possibly endure the strength of transition? I refer to these as emotional hurdles. They typically happen during active labor and again during transition. Many women want to flee from the situation whether it is by drugs, or actually checking out and going home! What is important to know is that they soon pass after a few contractions and she is able to continue on. You are especially vulnerable to the suggestions of the enemy at this time, so anticipate it and combat it with scripture.

This time in labor is very similar to the runner's block. If you know any long-distance runners, they might have explained to you this phenomenon. The runner's block is the point when the runner feels that they are completely exhausted and couldn't possibly take another step. They know, however, that if they continue past that emotional hurdle, they get a second wind and can go for another five miles.

Just as runners can achieve a second wind, laboring women can achieve it as well. There are observable times in women's births when they just want to give up. This is when she typically wants to have pain medication. Most of the women who go ahead with the pain medication either find out that the medication doesn't alleviate the pain entirely, or they find that they really didn't need it.

I have seen a few women who were totally satisfied with their medication experience. Most, however, said that if they had to do it over again, they would have waited a little while longer to see if they could make it without drugs. The most effective tool in getting past these rough emotional hurdles is simply recognizing them and knowing that in a few more contractions, a second wind is waiting.

It can be encouraging to hear yourself begin to want to give up, because then you know that you are progressing to the next phase of labor. Just knowing that in a few more contractions you will be able to regain control is very comforting. A great scripture reference is found in Isaiah 40:31 that says, "*but those who wait upon the Lord will renew their strength. They will soar on wings like eagles; they will walk and not be faint.*"

Meditations

1. As you are having a contraction, see the inside layer of your uterus. Try to see it loosening up and letting go. Then see the middle layer and the blood vessels. Picture them rich with blood that is supplying the baby with lots of oxygen. Next see the outer layer working hard to stretch the cervix. Lastly, envision your cervix as it opens during a contraction. Move back and forth between the different layers until you actually feel this working. Pray specifically that your uterus would work perfectly and in order. Pray that your cervix would remain supple and open, permitting each contraction to accomplishits work.

2. Imagine that you are a piece of seaweed that is attached to a rock at on the ocean floor. The current of the ocean moves the seaweed to and fro, and it yeilds to the motion, yet it is anchored to the rock. During a contraction, yeild to the force of the wave of strength your body is engaging it by letting go of all tension. Let go of everything that holds you, except for your Rock, Jesus Christ.

3. Picture a sweet rosebud that has been given to you. You place it in a glass of water so that it might bloom in due time. The rosebud represents the child that has been given to you, and the water represents the living water of peace the Jesus gives to us. We place our children in the living water that is within us, the peace that overcomes us when we are in trial. As we yield to God's design for nature, as we recognize that He designed a rose to open and bloom when it is ready, we also know that He formed us to open and bloom for the birth of our baby, not matter how long it takes. Let the living water flow from you, and be at peace and rest during this time.

4. Finally, picture the Lord Jesus Christ as he suffered on the cross. Remember how He asked God to take the cup from Him, but nevertheless, not His will but God's will be done. Picture every time He

took a breath, He had to lift Himself up so that He could inhale Crucifixion prevents respirations, ultimately suffocating the person when their legs were too weak to lift them, or were broken by the soldiers.

His nail-pierced feet had to elevate Him to breathe. As you breathe, remember His suffering and how He willingly endured that for us. Our light affliction lasts only a moment, and we too endure any discomfort for the joy set before us, that of receiving a new life in our arms when we have completed the work.

4. Prayer - As you feel a contraction coming, begin to say the following prayer, or come up with a new one for yourself.

"In the name of Jesus Christ, who I love and serve, I ask that my body would remain calm and completely relaxed. I pray for a quick birth, but not too quick to hurt my baby. I ask You for Your perfect timing, Lord. I give my body permission to open up and stretch to let my baby out in Your perfect timing, Lord."

Prayer is our direct line to the awesome power of the Lord. Think of it as a telephone wire and during your labor and delivery, you are able to communicate with Jesus and ask Him to intercede for you. Don't let a single contraction go by without praying, and when you pray, do it fervently with all of your heart. Acknowledge how great the Lord is and how thankful you are that you are in His arms of love, safe and sound, receiving this special gift of life into your family. Actually feel His warm arms around you as you talk to Him during a contraction. The Bible promises that if we draw near to Him, then He will draw near to us, and that whenever two or more are gathered in His name, He will be in their midst. Even if you are all alone while birthing, you are still two in number (you and your baby!) so rejoice in the fact that the Lord promises that He is in your midst and is waiting for you to reach out to Him so that you can enjoy His peace during labor.

5. Your Labor Partner - No woman should have to labor alone, we were designed to depend on each other. It is now known that women who have a doula with them during labor have more favorable memories of the birth, better outcomes, and healthier babies. Choose your labor partner carefully, making sure that they will be supportive and helpful to you. Many will want to witness the birth, but remember this is your time, and those who will be there with you should bring comfort to you, rather than you bringing entertainment to them. Consider bringing a doula with you and your husband; it will increase your odds for having a satisfying birth experience by leaps and bounds.

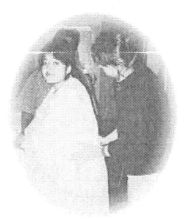

6.   Helpful positions   The positions you assume during childbirth are extremely important. Lying in bed the entire time without changing positions every hour is not necessarily a great idea. If you are able to get up out of bed, then you may want to try some of these positions that have been very useful for many women.

a. <u>Slow Dancing</u>

Slow dancing is a favorite among many women, because it allows them to be face to face with their partner while remaining in an upright position during the contraction. Please refer to the illustration to see how it is done and notice that her arms are dangling loose without needing to hold on to him. *It is important to rotate your hips in a circle, or a figure-eight, during the contraction.* This helps guide the baby's head lower into the pelvis.

If you have ever tried to force something into a small opening, you probably rotated it back and forth as you pushed on it to get it to go down further into the opening. This is the same principle. Babies heads often times do not fit just right through the pelvic opening, but by rotating your hips, you are gently coaxing the baby to drop down lower into the pelvis, helping labor along tremendously. Many women find that they will do this action instinctively during a contraction. Have your partner remind you each time, if you forget.

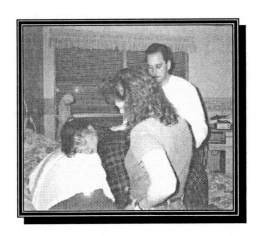

b. Birth Ball

The birth ball is a real nice way to remain upright while still being able to sit. Because it is inflated, it gives just enough to not put pressure on the tender perineum during a contraction. You will also be able to do hip rotations in this position. If you are having back labor, you may want to try the birth ball so that you can get into a semi-squat position which helps open your pelvis so that the baby can turn into the correct position. You can obtain a birth ball at www.cuttingedgepress.net. They are actually called exercise balls and have been used for physical therapy, but we use them at the hospital during childbirth. If you go to your local Big 5 sporting goods store and ask for a birth ball, they may possibly look at you a little funny! If you cannot afford one, contact the hospital that you will be birthing and ask if they have one already. If they don't have one and you purchase one yourself, you may consider donating yours after you have had your baby.

c. Anything Upright

Imagine your baby's head inside your uterus. If you are lying in bed, the weight of the baby's head is on the side or back of the uterus. Now if you were to stand up, gravity would cause the weight of the baby's head to shift and be placed down on the cervix. Because you are in an upright position, the weight of the baby's head helps the cervix to dilate faster than if you spent your entire labor in bed. If for some reason you are confined to bed, try lifting the head of the bed up so that you are in a semi-sitting position so that you can take advantage of gravity in order to speed things along.

Where is gravity?

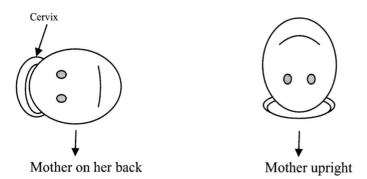

Mother on her back   Mother upright

When mom is upright, the gravity places the head directly on the cervix, and baby tends to assume a proper position. This speeds labor in and of itself. If a narcotic or epidural have been administered, and the mother must lay in bed continuously, the cervix must open by the power of the uterus only.

       d. <u>Water (Jacuzzi, shower, tub)</u>

       Many hospitals have at least one jacuzzi available for moms to get into while they are laboring. If you chose to get into the jacuzzi, do so after four centimeters because prior to that, it could slow down or stop labor. If you are unable to use the jacuzzi, then try using a shower or bathtub. The only other problem that I have seen with the jacuzzi is the fact that it is very difficult to get the mom out of it because she likes it so much!

Avoiding Back Labor

       Labor and delivery go much smoother when the baby is in the ideal position. This position is called "anterior occiput." The occiput is the back part of the head, the part that the Jewish men put their Yamica head coverings. The occiput needs to be applied to the cervix in a snug manner, covering it entirely so that it can act like a rolling pin on the cervix, pressing it thinner and helping it melt open the door that allows the passage of the baby.

       The occiput is a round area of the head, and can be somewhat applied to the cervix whether or not the baby's face is toward the pubic bone or the backbone. In order to understand anterior occiput and posterior occiput, it is first necessary to be able to orientate these two positions. The medical community has labeled the various areas of the body to limit the words needed for description and reference.

Anterior vs. posterior refers to the height or depth of a location on the body. If a person was laying on an exam table on their back, the anterior portion of their body would be that closest to the ceiling and the posterior would be that which was closest to the exam table. Therefore, the pubic bone would be considered anterior, while the tail bone would be considered posterior. A good way to remember posterior is that the backbone is similar to a post, which connects to the sacrum. It is important for the care provider to know which position the baby is facing, because if the baby is in the wrong position, labor can be lengthened and more complicated.

The care provider will check if the occiput is closer to the anterior part of the body, or the posterior. For example, if the baby's head is occiput anterior, the baby's face is against the tailbone and the occiput is against the pubic bone. In this position, the head passes through the pelvis with the smallest diameter. If the baby is in the posterior position, with the occiput against the sacrum and tailbone and the face against the pubic bone, the head not only presents a larger diameter, but cannot be applied to the cervix uniformly and so the "rolling pin" action is not as effective. On top of that, the occiput is hard and durable, not giving way at all, causing the infamous "back labor" that can be so difficult to cope with.

Preventing this position before labor and delivery has begun is definitely a wise thing to do. Practicing good pregnancy posture before the baby has "dropped" into the pelvis in the last weeks of pregnancy should help make things go even smoother. Keep in mind that this position occurs because the weight of the baby's back is heavier than his abdomen, so any position that puts the mother in a reclining state encourages the baby to flip around into the posterior position, much like a loose watch will invariably slide down with the face below the wrist. The common American couch, seat of a car, or chair at the computer desk puts the mother in a semi-reclining position that tempts the baby to slip into the posterior.

Good pregnancy posture is anything that gets you leaning forward. Watching television while leaning over your birth ball, sitting forward in your chair at the table and computer, and sleeping on your side at night are all good examples of proper positioning.

Occasionally it will happen that the baby is in the posterior position during labor. This can be suspected if the one or more of the following conditions exist:

1. Contractions hurt mostly in the lower back, just above the buttocks
2. The ache in the lower back does not fully disappear between contractions
3. The dilation of the cervix stalls for an extended period of time (usually around 5-6cm)
4. The care provider assesses the position of the baby's head based on the position of the fontanels (soft spots).

If the baby is suspected to be posterior, there are several things that the birth party can do in an attempt to encourage the baby to get into a more optimal position. It usually is very uncomfortable for mom, but if she is willing to invest some effort in helping the baby to get into a better spot, it will be easier for both her and her child in the long run. The pelvis is bony and space is limited down deep in the pelvis, so the idea is to either make more room down there for him to turn, or gently coax him out temporarily so that he can turn, or both. Maneuvers that have consistently helped other little people to get into the right position follow:

1. Knee-chest Position (most effective) – The mother gets on a soft surface and sits on her knees, crosses her arms and rests her chest on them so that her buttocks is higher than her shoulders. Gravity helps the baby out of the pelvis enough to get the uncomfortable bony pelvis off of his head and to flip around because of the weight of his back. Ten minutes in this position usually does the trick, but more time may be needed for babies who are deeper in the pelvis. VARIATION: This can also be done (less effectively) in the hands and knees position combining it with hip rotations and hip tucks. The back should be guarded so as not to allow the spine to drop below the level of the shoulders to prevent strain.

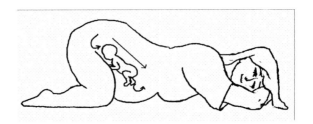

2. Abdominal Lift – Some have found it helpful to lift the abdomen up **during** a contraction to encourage the baby out of the pelvis enough to turn. This combined with the following belly dance can be very effective as well.
3. The Belly Dance – By the time the mother has gone into labor, her body has allowed the joints to become much more flexible and moveable. If she rotates the hips **during** a contraction, it will help flex the bones around, encouraging the baby to turn. It is similar to trying to stuff a large item into a hole. You twist and turn as it goes in, helping it along…
4. Stair Climbing – Much like belly dancing, stair climbing can rotate the hips enough to encourage a better position.

Pain relief - Posterior babies can be tasking on the birth party, and any father whose wife had a back labor can tell you that his arms where like noodles the next day after the birth! The mother will need constant counter pressure on her lower back to relieve the discomfort of the head of the baby pressing against it. The area that needs counter-pressure is the lower segment of the spine, directly on the sacrum itself. The sacrum is just above the "crack" of the buttocks, and appears as an inverted triangle-shape indentation. This is typically the exact location of discomfort for a mother with a posterior baby, and she will need firm and constant pressure against it.

To apply counter pressure, make a fist and place the flat part of your fingers against the sacrum. Inquire of the mother how firm she would like you to press, as sometimes just a light stroking is better. More often than not, the mom wants full-strength and constant pressure applied in order to achieve relief.

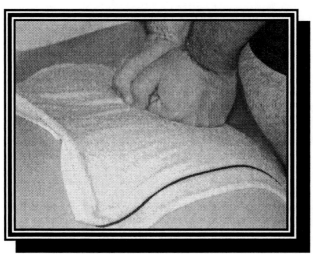

Taken by Maureen Johnston & Monique Micallef

In addition to counter pressure, try using a cold or hot pack on the sacrum, use items such as a tennis ball, massager, rolling pin, rice sock, etc. Some couples have had success having the father get down close to the belly and tell the baby to turn into the right position. The most important thing is prayer, of course, before and during labor that in the name of Jesus, the baby would get into the proper positioning so that the labor and birth will be normal and more comfortable.

Pushing Techniques

For the birth of your child, you are blessed with the awesome opportunity to actively bring forth your baby into the world. The movies portray it as an event that takes place with sterile gloves, face shields, scissors, needles, and the like. For some, this is what needs to take place in order to manage a complicated situation or a cesarean delivery. For the normal birthing situation, however, most hospitals allow you to take a more active role in the delivery. The sterile atmosphere then turns into a more cozy, family environment.

Premature Urge to Push

Women usually remember this time in labor more vividly than any other. They are told that their cervix is not dilated to ten centimeters yet and they cannot push. The urge is so strong that it

133

would be like telling your child to stop vomiting. It is nearly impossible to keep from it. The best technique that I can share with you for this one is panting. It is fairly simple; you just lift your head up as high as it will go and pant rapidly. Be careful, however, or you'll hyperventillate! To prevent this, pant as if you are blowing out a birthday candle and say the word "puhh, puhh, puhh, ..." There is something about lifting your head and panting that keeps you from being able to push. I would say it is helpful for about 90 percent of the women, but there is always that one or two who just cannot stop pushing.

It may increase your incentive to resist the urge to push by knowing that if you push before it is time, the cervix could begin to swell and actually get smaller in diameter. This can actually land you in the operating room for a cesarean. If you are 8-9 centimeters and you have the overwhelming desire to push, many nurses will let you do little grunts and this might actually help the cervix to continue to dilate. It is hard to know what is best in this situation. By pushing, you may help the cervix or you may cause it to swell. This is a decision best left to the medical team to make the call. Remember Philipians 4:19 which says "I can do all things through Christ who strengthens me."

No Urge to Push

This situation is a little more difficult to manage. First off, you should know that it is perfectly normal to have a 15 – 30 minute break between first stage and second stage labor. It is a little regrouping and resting session for you before the work begins. However, not all women experience this. If you are completely dilated and having contractions but no urge to push, and it has been longer than half an hour, consider getting into a position that will get the baby's head as low in the pelvis as possible. A good supported squat is ideal for this.

If, after you have tried various positions and still have not gotten the urge, you may want to ask yourself if there is a hidden fear that is unresolved. Many women are fearful of tearing their perineum. Others are afraid that they will not be a good parent, or may not be ready for parenthood. The mind is very powerful and capable of halting all efforts of the body to birth the baby. Our loving Father is able to cast out all of our fears by His power, not ours, and so we rest in that knowledge and ask Him to give us the strength to finish the task.

Some women have unresolved abuse issues that may hinder second stage. Whether it was physical or sexual, they were out of control of their bodies then, and they feel out of control once again. Many do well, but for most, they feel as though the abuse is happening all over again. The good news is that first and foremost, if any man be in Christ he is a new creation. This includes the girls too. We are a new creature and can let go of the created body of the past.

Secondly, the Lord has been gracious enough to give us a measure of control over this situation. We may not be in control of our bodies, but we can claim control over our mind. Either we can allow Satan to once again come in and destroy this precious moment, or we can be free in Christ and remain quiet and at peace. Satan wants us to relive the experience, being violated once again. Jesus Christ, on the other hand, wants us to be in control of the birth of this child, and we do that by the Holy Spirit. One of the fruits of the spirit is peace, and if we abide in the Holy Spirit, He will bring this fruit about in our life during this most precious time. Where there once was pain as a punishment, there is now pain with a purpose. This time, we get a lovely little present to take home with us to treasure!

Different Pushing Styles

The most natural way to push is how you will feel that you need to push. For some, this comes automatically and it is the safest way to deliver your baby. You will breathe when you need to breathe, and push when you need to push. For how long, you ask? A normal second stage labor takes anywhere from one push to 2 hours. Depending on the Doctor, you may need to have more active coaching if you have been pushing for 30 – 45 minutes without much progress.

Many first-timers will need some type of coaching during this stage. If you are a newbie at it and not sure how it's done, it is okay for the staff to direct you on where to push and for how long. I need to mention that there are times when it is necessary to get the baby delivered quickly and the staff will actively coach you to deliver if the baby is compromised. It is important to note, however, that this type of active coaching during a normal birth can actually cause a decrease of oxygen to your baby and create a situation that would not have happened otherwise. This is the type of pushing where you see them taking a huge breath and holding it as their face turns purple and the nurse makes her hold it for the count of ten.

Directions for Normal Pushing

When your cervix is completely dilated, it is time to push the baby out and into your arms. You will know this time is nearing because you begin to feel as though you have to go to the bathroom and have a bowel movement. This happens because the baby's head is pressing against the nerve in your rectum that normally alerts you that there is stool to be passed. This pressure from the head is very intense and builds until you have no other choice but to bear down.

As your contractions shift to this kind of sensation, you will not need as much concentration to remain relaxed. You become more alert and participate more in the conversations around the room. Again, many women are very relieved during the second stage and report that it actually "feels better" to push.

Remember that because you are pushing, you may be holding your breath for an extended period of time. It is important, then, to make sure that before you start your push, to take a deep breath of air first to ensure that your baby gets enough oxygen. As you bear down, it is better to go ahead and exhale your air with vocal efforts. The vocal sounds should be with an open throat and a low tone. A tight voice equals a tight birth canal, and can take away from the work of your delivery. This instinctual grunting is wonderful, as long as all the effort is below the waist. I have seen a lady push for five hours, with the first three hours being all voice. She redirected her efforts to her bottom, and when she got the hang of it, did very nicely.

Since a contraction lasts from 60 – 90 seconds, you should be able to get three pushes in before it is time to rest. Each time you push from your bottom (as if you are having a bowel movement), you move the baby closer to birth. The baby inches down little by little, stretching the vaginal tissue gently so that it won't tear. When you push, the baby's head comes down a little, and when you take a breath before your next push in the same contraction, the baby can slip back up into the canal. This is very normal an is God's design to help the birth canal stretch and open little by little.

136

Preventing A Tear

The best way to prevent a tear is to be in a position that facilitates the birth. If a person is laying flat on their back, then they are pushing the baby out and up, against gravity. The little head pushes right against the perineum and increases the risk of a serious tear. Squatting, on the other hand, allows the baby to come down in the angle best conducive to gravity.

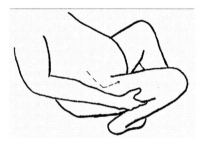

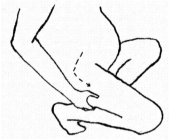

Semi-reclining   Squatting

Other things that can be done to prevent a tear:

~ Proper hydration
~ Warm compresses to the perineum during second stage
~ Non-petroleum based oil to the perineum during second stage
~ An open and relaxed perineum during a push. Allowing the bottom to just drop down and not resist the push will help prevent a tear.

Delivery

Many are surprised to find out that they can actually deliver the body of the baby themselves. Most assume that the doctor will do it and hand you the baby. But if your birth is complication-free and you are in a good position, you may want to reach down and hold the baby under his arms and deliver the him yourself. Even the squeamish can do this during the excitement of the moment. It is a beautiful gift to be able to say that you truly brought this child into the world.

Not all will have the presence of mind to reach down and retrieve their child. Many will be so exhausted that they are not sure if the baby's head is even out yet. For this person I say, take heart. You are transformed within seconds after your baby's birth and as you come around, your exhaustion shall be exchanged for joy as you gaze into this new little life's eyes. Even still, many women do not feel that initial feeling of joy right after the birth, and that is okay too. Bonding takes a lifetime and, Lord willing, a lifetime you will have.

Clamping the Cord

A controversial subject is that of claping and cutting the cord. When to do it? I always ask myself, "If a woman was by herself and she delivered her child, would she immediately grab something to clamp the cord with?" Of course not. The cord continues pulsating for many minutes after the baby has been delivered. This is providing your baby with much needed oxygen, just in case breathing has not gotten off to a good start. Also, there is a volume of blood that is in the cord that returns to the baby before it stops pulsing. Keep in mind that if a complication arises, the care provider will clamp and cut the cord automatically and take the baby to the warming cart where the specialists can begin to fix the problem.

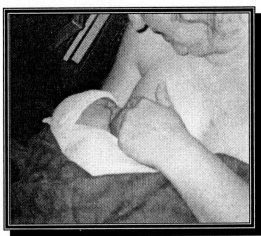

Courtesy of Lori Lee

1. Practice Abdominal Breathing while listening to soothing worship music.

2. Try the hands/knees position, as well as the knees/chest position. Have your partner give you a back rub in this position.

3. Time the length of a typical contraction to get a feel for how long it will be lasting.

4. Start thinking about a birth plan.

5. End the evening with slow dancing. The two of you, and your baby, can pamper each other…why not?

Chapter Ten
Your Bondservant For Birth

Believe it or not, there are those who passionately desire to help you when your baby comes into this world. Much of their life is devoted to seeing women *enjoy* their birth and early parenting, doing their best to help thwart a negative experience. Although God has appointed some to be overseers of the clinical aspects of the event, He also has set a fire in the hearts of some women just to buddy up with you and serve your every want and need during labor and delivery. Acting as the guardian of your memories, she truly is your bondservant for birth.

In Exodus 21, Moses explains to us what a doulos, or bondservant, is. Different from a purchased slave, the bondservant offers his life-time service by his own will, out of his love for the master. This applies to our dear Lord because He has willingly devoted Himself to be the servant of God and all of humanity because of his love for His Father. It applies to His redeemed people as well, who choose to serve the Master with all of their heart, soul, and mind for all of their lives. And finally, the female version of the word for bondservant (doula) has been adopted to refer to a woman who chooses to become the servant of the expectant family during pregnancy, labor, delivery, and the postpartum period.

The title and position of the *doula* is accepted by the medical community as one who comes alongside the family during the transition to parenthood, acting as their maternity care planner, remaining with them throughout labor and delivery, and debriefing them after the birth. Although her training in pregnancy and childbirth may be extensive, she offers no clinical service to the mother or the baby such as internal exams, fetal heart rate monitoring, or taking vital signs. She does offer supplemental childbirth education, a responsible look at birth decisions and their effects/consequences, as well as physical comfort measures and educated encouragement during the birth. She is trained in traditional ways to handle the difficult birth, using very effective techniques to facilitate a more normal and faster birth.

Because of her very specific training, she also focuses on the emotional aspects of labor and delivery that are typically not taught to clinical care providers. She is trained in successful breastfeeding techniques, postpartum and newborn issues, and godly parenting (if she is Christian).

It is not surprising that the act of serving a woman during birth, which is God's model in all aspects of life, can bring many wonderful and impressive benefits. Medical scientists are now documenting as fact what the Bible has been teaching us all along - that there is joy involved when we put others' needs before our own and serve them with a willing heart. These joys are manifested in childbirth by way of improved medical and social outcomes, and the benefits are numerous and far reaching.

Twenty Great Reasons to Have A Doula [1]

1. The benefit of uninterrupted personal care.
2. Fewer cesarean sections, by up to 50%.
3. Shorter labors by up to 25%.
4. Fewer requests for epidurals by up to 60%.
5. Fewer requests for IV pain killers by up to 40%.
6. Pitocin augmentation reduction by 30%.
7. Need for forceps reduced by 40%.
8. Reduced maternal fevers.
9. Reduced pain at 24 hours postpartum.
10. Reduced postpartum hemorrhage.
11. Greater success with breastfeeding.
12. Greater satisfaction with the birth process, the hospital, and staff.
13. Greater satisfaction with their partner.
14. Better bonding with the baby immediately after birth.
15. More affectionate interactions with baby.
16. Shorter hospital stays for the baby.
17. Fewer admissions to the neonatal intensive care unit.
18. Decreased incidence of postpartum depression.
19. Decreased health problems with the infant at six weeks.
20. Dramatically reduced medical costs.

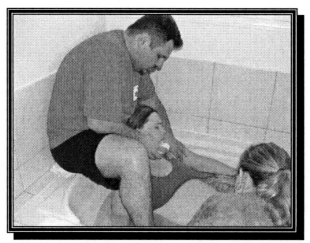

Taken by Maureen Johnston & Monique Micallef

Why not just have a friend or relative act as your doula? This is a valid question, and has been explored by medical researchers recently. The question is posed as to why the professional doula would be needed on the obstetrical team. Surprisingly, there are two solid and scientific reasons why doula care exceeds the benefits of acquaintance care at the birth.

1. Although the presence of the family and friends at the birth was shown to be valued, the outcome of the birth was unaffected.[2]
2. Nurses were shown to have a positive effect for the mother, however the uninterrupted doula quality support given by nurses was reluctantly rare or non-existent.[3]

It is true that having a doula with you and your partner during delivery can enhance your experience greatly, as research has firmly shown. You may enjoy even greater benefit if the personality of the doula is a good match with yours. A recent study[4] has suggested that the selection of a compatible supporter is an important aspect of receiving the maximum benefit from doula care.

Because personalities and beliefs of each person are different, it is important to interview several doula candidates to ensure the best match. There are many approaches to doula care, and it is important to understand them so that you can ask the doula how she performs her duties during the interview. In an attempt to outline the various styles, the nuances of the profession have been separated into different categories for you and your doula to examine.

You can learn about each style so that you will have an idea of what you are looking for before the first visit, and she can describe to you which of these styles fit her the most accurately. Keep in mind, each doula is unique and she may oscillate from one characteristic to another depending on the circumstances of the birth.

The Cost of A Doula

As a rule of thumb, doulas spend about 30 -50 working hours with their clients, and anticipate being on call for the two weeks prior to the due date and for two weeks after (up to 672 hours on call). Most doulas have been to some type of formal training and have a financial investment in their certification. They are considered a paraprofessional, and treat their work like a business. To be a quality doula, one must be able to drop everything at once when the phone call comes in, making it difficult to be gainfully employed at a typical job. In addition, her work often prevents her family from being able to enjoy a trip to the beach or lake, and when she is called in, it is for an unknown amount of time. This can be taxing on her family and marriage, and for this reason, it is strongly suggested that the doula be paid according to this loving sacrifice that she so passionately makes.

The cost of doula services spreads to both extremes, with some doing all of their work voluntarily, to others charging lofty fees that exceed $1500. The cost of doula services depends on several factors:

1. The economic condition of your community.
2. The experience of your doula.
3. The services that your doula will provide.
4. Whether or not your doula works within a triad or group of doulas.
5. Whether or not your insurance will cover the expense

No one should be denied the service of a doula based on ability to pay. Most, if not all, doulas will charge on a sliding scale or will take barter. Many junior doulas are willing to offer services at reduced or no cost to gain experience. And most brand new doulas will pay you to let them come to your birth! This of course is not required, and is said in jest, but it *is* the attitude and fervent passion that is in the heart of the women God has called to be His birth maidservants.

Locating A Doula

Almost every community has at least one working doula, and many areas are saturated with the service. The idea has become increasingly more popular, making it easier to find someone nearby. As time passes, Christian doulas are becoming more prevalent as well. There are several resources that will assist you in finding that right person for your birth.

1. www.ChristianChildbirth.org
2. www.atfm.com
3. www.christianbirth.org
4. www.cappa.net
5. www.dona.org
6. www.childbirthsolutions.com/doulafinder/index.php
7. www.childbirth.org
8. www.birthpartners.com
9. www.birthingnaturally.net
10. Call your local childbirth educator.
11. Ask your care provider.
12. Ask your local midwife

The doula might seem like the newest member of the birthing team, but she is actually the oldest. Throughout time, women have been helping other women have babies. Now that the idea is being revisited, we are finding out that she may be the most important player on the obstetrical team when it comes to the comfort and satisfaction of birth. Be encouraged to find and hire a doula, you will cherish her!

References:
1. J Womens Health Gend Based Med 1999 Dec;8(10):1257-64
2. J Psychosom Obstet Gynaecol 1993 Mar;14(1):1-15
3. JAMA 2002 Sep 18;288(11):1373-81
4. Curationis 1995 Dec;18(4):77-80

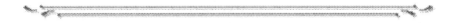

Bible Study Discussion

1. How many of you will be using a doula?

2. Do you have a list of doula names and phone numbers to share with the group?

3. Are there any concerns you have with using a doula?

4. Do you have any testimonies to share regarding the use of a doula?

5. What part of this chapter stands out to you?

Chapter Eleven
Prayers and Meditations

I would encourage you to write your own meditations as you move through your pregnancy. Choose a pretty journal from the bookstore and keep it primarily for prayers to the Lord during this time. It will be a cherished heirloom for generations to come after you. Here are some prayers and meditations for you to join together with me and other ladies around the world in common agreement and supplication. It is wonderful to know that we can all join in one voice on behalf of our children!

Late Pregnancy

Father, my heart rejoices over the work that You have done. My pregnancy is nearing completion and I am anticipating the beauty of my child. Lord, let every minute that I spend in these last days be given to You, so that Your strength would be absorbed by every breath that I take for me and my baby. Lord, although I may be uncomfortable for a moment, I know this joy will last a lifetime. I look to You for patience, God, so that my baby can grow inside me for each precious day that You have chosen to give us together before we separate and become two. Lord, only You know my child's hour to be born, and help me to honor that day and not be tempted to take control over what day that will be. Lord, if it is necessary, help me to place my child in the hands of the medical professionals, and I ask You to direct their thoughts and actions so that they would be the best for my baby. If everything is normal, Lord, I surrender to Your will and your timing; for only You know the day and the hour. You are on the throne and You reign in my life, God almighty, and I sit and wait for You. Not my will, Lord, but Yours, and Yours alone. You are holy and I trust You and submit to Your ways. Praise Your name Lord, God! Be glorified in this birth. In Jesus' name, Amen

Post Date

Abide in my heart, Lord. I am ready to bear this fruit, and You said that if we abide in You, that we would bear much fruit! I know this is regarding spiritual things, Lord, but I jest and rejoice in this scripture, knowing that we cannot bear fruit by ourselves, so we seek You and Your divine providence in this time of waiting. Lord, I ask that my baby would be healthy, and that this time within me would be adding strength to his little body. God, I wait for You and Your will and timing. Search my heart, O God, and see if there would be any root of fear there. Lord let the fear run through my closed fist like sand, God. Even though I may hold on to it tightly, Your word says You take fear away from me in 1 John 4:18, and so I believe that promise.

I also pray that my baby would get into a perfect position and prepare to come, in the name of Jesus Christ. Blessed is the one who puts their trust in You, and I do just that God. Direct my paths on how these overdue days should be spent. Lord help me remember that a normal pregnancy is from 38 – 42 weeks. Lord, You suffered greatly that day on the cross, more than any man has ever endured. Knowing that You did this for me helps me to endure a few more days. Lord, if my baby is not okay, then help me to be confident in my medical team, knowing that they can help. Lord, bring this baby the way that You have   designed,
In Jesus' precious name, Amen

Robert and Stephanie's Labor

Taken by Maureen Johnston & Monique Micallef

Onset of Labor

God, I know that You can do all things, and I ask that You make it very apparent that my labor has started. I have waited for this day a long time, and I desire peace when it comes. Place a hedge of protection around my heart so that the enemy would not have a foothold to begin the cycle of fear and uncertainty. Your waters replenish my soul, Lord, and I pray that your Spirit would rain down on me the day my labor begins. Help me to seek your peace, and not the peace of the world. As I breathe in Your Spirit, I drink in Your presence and it radiates throughout my body, bringing total tranquility. I feel the glow of your Holy Spirit surrounding me, warm and holy. The glory of the work you have done shines on me, and I am Your child. Let not my heart be troubled and let not my heart be afraid. I receive Your love and Your peace that You have left for me. I am anxious for nothing, and Your peace that passes all understanding is guarding my heart against the darts of the enemy. I can hear voices inside my head trying to discourage me, Lord, but I ask You to cast them out as far as the East is from the West. You're my best friend, Lord, come and fly with me as I soar with You high above the world and focus only on You and my baby. Stay with me this day, God.

In your Son's beautiful name, Amen

Early Labor

I lift my eyes toward Heaven, and look for You this day. I know that You are with me God, and I love You. Wrap Your arms around me as I feel my baby stretch and turn into a perfect position. You are my shepherd Jesus, and I look to You for guidance now. Show me what you would have me do right now that would be the best. If it is night time, help me rest between contractions. If it is daytime, God, help me remain upright and active, but conserving strength. I can do all things through You, because You strengthen me. I will not fear what lies ahead, but will accept it, God. I know that I am fearfully and wonderfully made, and that You are God of everything. I rejoice this very moment in You, Jesus. I thank you for Your loving kindness and longsuffering. Help me to love my child in this way: to be patient and longsuffering for the good of my child.

Early Labor Meditation

I love You, I praise You, I worship You, and I adore You. I want to give glory to Your name, You are my song. Be my strength, guard my soul, control my mind, oh best friend. You died, so that I could live. Live through me now Jesus. I love You...

Active Labor

Lord, thank You for each contraction that you have given me. I know that each one will bring me closer to my child's first breath. Lord, show my child the way to come out, and see the world that You have made. Lord, I know that You rest not during this time. I know that You always were, are now, and always will be on the throne. Your dominion is forever, and I can almost hear angels singing, "Holy, holy, holy is the Lord God almighty, who was and is, and is forevermore."

I give my body permission to open up and let my baby out. I release all tension, for I know that it is not of You but of the enemy. Fear and tension are branches that bear no fruit, and I know that if I allow that fear to take root, that I may not be able to bear the fruit of my womb. So then, I ask You to prune that branch of fear, and throw it to the fire to be burned. I cannot do it on my own, Lord, but I know that You can. Bring me back to a state of deep rest in You, Lord, and please take away all distractions so that I can hear Your waves of comfort rush over me. I know that this is a time of great vulnerability to the attack of Satan, and I pray against that in Jesus' name. I understand that if I remain in You and in Your peace, I will find new strength to continue on. I will not believe the lie that says that it will get twice as hard from this point. Lord, I am pressed but not crushed. I have made it this far, Lord, take me the rest of the way. You are a sun and a shield, Lord. You give us grace and glory, and no good thing will You withhold from those of us who put our trust in You. Blessed are you, Lord! You are my God and my strength! Be with me now, overcome any evil thoughts, You have complete control over me.

Shield my heart and my mind, and give your grace to me now, in Jesus' name, Amen

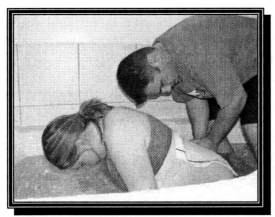

Taken by Maureen Johnston & Monique Micallef

Meditation for Active Labor

Blessed is the one that puts their trust in Him. Renew a right spirit within me, Jesus. You replenish my soul, I drink You in and breathe out anything unholy. Please forgive all that I hold, and take charge right now. I need You right now, Lord. Help me to be calm. I hide beneath Your wings, and cling to You in a peaceful rest. Focus my thoughts on my baby, and let every decision that I make be borne of You, for the good of Your child. I love my baby, God, and I dedicate this time to You. My thoughts are Yours God... My thoughts are Yours, God... My thoughts are Yours God... replenish my soul.

Transition

Do you see this woman, Jesus? Here I am, Lord, hard pressed but not crushed, nor abandoned. I receive your peace, now more than ever. I keep a smile on my face, Lord, because now is the time before everything changes. These contractions will be productive, and every breath belongs to You. I refuse to give into the thoughts that have their origin in fear. I rejoice greatly in the fact that my child will be here soon. I am not afraid of becoming a parent, Lord, I know that You will direct my paths. I tremble, Lord, but let me tremble in the power of your creation. Lord, the whole world trembled when you said, "It is finished." You suffered so greatly, but you willingly did so, for the joy set before you, and you endured the cross so that we might live. Lord, let me endure this time so that my child might be born and begin life outside the womb.

I realize that any tension at all right now will only delay that moment, and I certainly don't want to get stuck in this stage of labor. Let me go deep within myself and see your face there before me. If I weep, let it be as a woman who is longing for her child. Let me wash your feet with my tears and wipe them with my hair. I cannot anoint your head with oil, but let me sing you a love song to anoint you with my love. If I cry out, let it be unto you in rejoicing. If I cling to something, let it be as one who is clinging to you in her most desperate hour. Then let me release my grip in total trust and belief that you will complete the work that you have started in me.

You say you are the Alpha and the Omega, the beginning and the end. I am praying for the end of this work, so that I may hold my little baby on my breast. Open the eyes of my heart Lord, that I might see you now. Open the door of my womb, Lord, that I might see my child. Father God, free my child into my arms.

In your Son's name, Amen

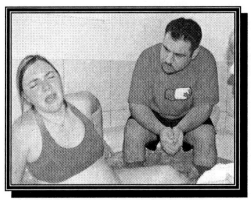

Taken by Maureen Johnston & Monique Micallef

Meditation for Transition

Father God, in the name of Jesus Christ, (who I love and adore) cause me to be completely relaxed and tranquil in You. I surrender all..., I surrender all..., take my life, I give it to you. Lead me beside still water, restore my soul. Let me be a testimony right now, of your great love. Do not withhold anything good, pour out your blessing on me. Open the floodgates of my strength, which comes from you... I work in great peace that many cannot understand. It is by You only, You only…., You only! Praise God!

Second Stage (Pushing)

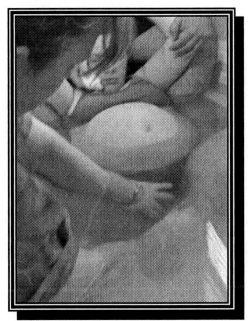

Taken by Maureen Johnston & Monique Micallef

Renew my strength with every breath you give me. Spirit, fall on me like the rain. Come down from the Heavens and hold my hand. I worship you right now with all my heart, strength, soul, and mind. Direct my thoughts, and show me the way to birth my child. You give us direction, Lord, when we ask. I wait on You, Lord. I am not rushed, friend Jesus, but wait for You. I drink in the oxygen that you made, and it nourishes my child as I yield to the force of life. I let my inner parts drop low with warmth and supple heat, not resisting the feeling. I am perfectly made to do this, Lord, Creator of my body.

Lord let everything go smoothly and according to Your design. If I need help, let skilled and patient hands show me the way. I am not afraid to open my eyes and look upon the face that you created inside of me. I long to hold a little hand and help birth a new love of my life. I pray that this little person, being born right now, will know you intimately. I am caught up in the mystery of this moment. You have

placed a banner over me, and on it is written "LOVE." I love the little person inside of me and long to see its wrinkled little face! My heart is swelling with joy and anticipation. Lord, if for some reason I am not feeling joy, Lord, I know that you will fill my heart in due time, and I am at peace with this. Give us this day our new child…, your child.
I rest in Your love and in Your life…, live through us this day.
In Jesus' name, Amen

Meditation For Second Stage

You are the true vine, and I am a branch of you. I allow you to abide in me, and I am abiding in you, so that I will bear your fruit this day. It is harvest time, Lord, we receive your child.

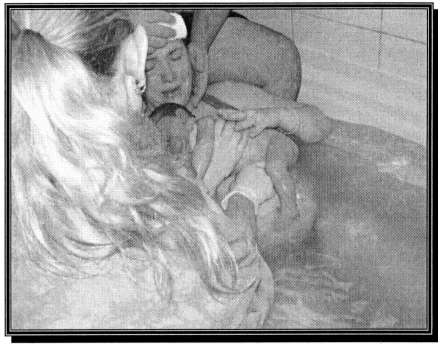

Taken by Maureen Johnston & Monique Micallef

Bible Study Discussion

1. Do you have any personal mediations you would like to share?

2. Do you have any personal testimonies you would like to share?

3. Perhaps you might watch another positive birth video tonight.

4. What part of this chapter stands out to you?

5. Spend time in prayer together…

Chapter Twelve
Helpful Scripture Passages

I would encourage you write down these scriptures on index cards so that you will have them available for the birth. There is nothing more powerful than the Word of God! Don't forget them…

James 4:7 – 8

> *Submit yourselves to God. Resist the devil, and he*
> *will flee from you.*

In the book of James, we are given the keys on how to overcome temptation and sin in our life. James says that we are to resist Satan's attempts of suggestive thoughts in our mind. There is a second part of the prescription, however. James goes on to say, *"Draw near to God, and He will come near to you."*

If you are finding that you are trying everything to resist temptation, but are unsuccessful, you may want to ask yourself if you are near to the Lord. The Lord is eternal and unchanging. His love for us is unending and unconditional. If we feel that God is far from us, we may want to ask ourselves if it is *we* who are not close to Him.

I once heard a pastor tell a story that illustrates this situation perfectly. There was an older couple who were driving in their truck; he in the drivers seat, and she across the bench. The wife said to the husband, "How come we never sit by each other any more? When we were young, we used to sit side by side together everywhere we went. Now it just isn't the same." Her husband looked over to her and said, "I didn't move."

Isn't it true? God doesn't move. When we feel that our relationship with the Lord just isn't the same anymore and we don't feel the presence of God, we might hear Him say, "I didn't move!" So James 4:8 is an excellent scripture for us to know that to better resist Satan, we must return to a close relationship with the Lord.

Jeremiah 29:13

You will seek me and find me when you seek me with all of your heart. I will be found by you, declares the Lord, and will bring you back from captivity.

There is a wonderful promise in Jeremiah that says that if you seek the Lord with all of your heart, *you will find Him.* We must ask ourselves if we are in captivity to fear. If so, we are given the solution and that is to seek the Lord with all of our heart. Once He is found by us, he will deliver us.

The Lord is a loving God and desires to bless His children. His thoughts toward us each day are as numerous as the grains of sand on the seashore. Earlier in Jeremiah 29:11 it says, *"For I know the thoughts that I think toward you, says the Lord, thoughts of peace and not of evil, to give you a future and a hope."* It is true that He wants to bless us through His son Jesus Christ. Many people think that God is a white-haired angry judge that is waiting to strike someone down with a lightening bolt. And that is just what Satan would have you to think. But by believing this scripture in Jeremiah, we know that the Lord desires to bless us, not to blast us! May you continue to seek Him with all of your heart.

Psalm 27:1- 3

The Lord is my light and my salvation; whom shall I fear? The Lord is the strength of my life; of whom shall I be afraid? When the wicked came against me to eat up my flesh, my enemies and foes, they stumbled and fell. Though an army should encamp against me, my heart shall not fear, though war should rise up against me, in this I will be confident.

We need not be afraid of the wicked one during labor and delivery. In fact, we can stand firm in the promises of God that He will deliver us from our enemy. With God's power, we can approach labor with great confidence!

Philippians 4:13

I can do all things through Christ who strengthens me.

During late pregnancy and childbirth, it is easy to want to give up and feel as though we are unable to continue on. Here is a scripture that we can tuck away in our hearts for those moments when we don't have the strength. We know that Jesus Christ will *give* us the strength to do all things, including birth.

It is perfectly normal for a woman to be seized with panic for a short period or part of her labor. It might be wise to expect that at some point in the labor, Satan will try to come in with an exceedingly strong arsenal of doubt and weariness as an attempt to begin the process of unnatural pain. The good news is that He who is in you is stronger than the one who is in the world. It is not by your own strength that you overcome these attacks, but by the hand of the Lord.

Philippians 4:6

Do not be anxious about anything, but in everything, by prayer and petition, with thanksgiving, present your requests to God.

Here it is. It is a command that we are not to be anxious about *anything,* including childbirth. Instead, we are to ask God for help with a thankful heart. Attitude is critical!

Proverbs 3:5 - 6

Trust in the Lord with all of your heart and lean not on your own understanding; in all your ways acknowledge Him, and He will direct your paths.

Our understanding tells us birth should be painful and something to fear. Our media, friends, family, and co-workers all have something to say about how difficult it is to give birth, and we even tell ourselves that. But we are commanded to not trust in our own understanding, but to lean on the Lord. We are also told to acknowledge Him in all of our ways, so we are to acknowledge Him in our birth as well. That means knowing that He is the author and finisher of our lives as well as our child's. We ought to submit to Him and allow Him to work His perfect love in this situation.

1 John 4:18

> *There is no fear in love. But perfect love casts out all fear because fear has to do with torment.*

In our own efforts, we may not be able to overcome the fear of birth, but God is perfect and it is His perfect love that can cast out fear for us. We have to let Him take it from us when we are unable.

Fear is from Satan, who wants to torment us. How many women do we know who have been tormented with thoughts of despair and guilt while giving birth? Ask Him to cast out that fear and He will; He promised that He would.

II Timothy 1:7

> *For God did not give us the spirit of fear, but a spirit of power, of love, and of self control.*

The fear we have is not from the Lord. We have to ask Him for the spirit that He gave us; the comfort of the Holy Spirit. The spirit of self-control is given to us by God as a gift and we can utilize it. Childbirth is a wonderful time to use our God-given self-control.

John 14:27

> *Peace I leave with you; my peace I give you. I do not give as the world gives. Do not let your hearts be troubled and do not be afraid.*

We can enjoy a peace that was given to us by Christ. His peace is much different than the peace given by earthly things. He says that He does not give as the world gives. How does the world give peace to birthing families? Ask the Lord to give you *His* peace during this time. See if He does not pour out a blessing on you that you would never have guessed could happen.

Jeremiah 1:5

Before I formed you in the womb I knew you, before you were born I set you apart.

We are set apart from the rest of the world. We are strangers and pilgrims to this world and many would consider us "crazy" to want to have a Christ-centered childbirth. But what a powerful testimony given when even in the most difficult birth, we can still have joy and give praise, honor, and glory to our God.

Romans 12:2

Do not conform any longer to the pattern of this world, but be transformed by the renewing of your mind.

We need to renew our minds when it comes to childbirth. We have been taught worldly things about childbirth and so it is written in scripture to let that go and renew your mind to a new way of thinking. Having a less painful, shorter childbirth *IS* possible! In fact, according to Judith Goldsmith in her book Childbirth Wisdom, the world average length of labor is four hours, not twelve hours like it is here in the Western world. It would be interesting to know why that is...

Psalm 34:4

I sought the Lord and He answered me; He delivered me from all my fears.

The psalmist acknowledged that it was not by his own strength that he could overcome fear, but he was delivered by God. It was the Lord's responsibility to be the deliverer, and it was the psalmist's responsibility to just seek the Lord. Our polite Savior waits quietly for us to seek Him, and when we do, He hears and is faithful to deliver us.

Isaiah 40:31

But they that wait upon the LORD shall renew their strength; they shall mount up with wings as eagles; they shall run, and not be weary; and they shall walk, and not faint." (KJV)

This verse can be applied to many instances in pregnancy and birth. We live in an instant-gratification society, and we are very pampered by what the world has to offer us. As Christians, when everything is normal, we can confidently seek the Lord for our comfort first. He promises us that those who wait for Him will be strengthened when we are weary. Pregnancy and birth carry with them many opportunities to grow in patience and perseverance!

James 5:10 – 11

Brothers, as an example of patience in the face of suffering, take the prophets who spoke in the name of the Lord. As you know, we consider blessed those who have persevered. You have heard of Job's perseverance and have seen what the Lord finally brought about. The Lord is full of compassion and mercy.

Yes, Job endured much suffering and loss, but he received it from the Lord, and in the end, the Lord restored everything to Job; even more than he had before. God is a good accountant, and if He requires suffering from us, He is faithful to restore us and even bless us with even more happiness. The mindset of the Christian isn't to completely escape suffering, but to persevere through it.

Psalm 1:1

Blessed is the man who does not walk in the counsel of the wicked or stand in the way of sinners or sit in the seat of mockers.

This basically says that we should not listen to the advice of the ungodly, whomever they might be. If someone is giving you advice that you have not asked for, or they are offering frightening stories, you are blessed if you do not count them as a worthy source of information. Even further, this scripture refers to the man who does not even sit in the seat of mockers. That is to say that we are not to even keep company with this type of person. We have enough trouble trying to resist the negative thoughts in our own head without having to accept negative thoughts from others!

2 Timothy 3:16

All scripture is God-breathed, and useful for teaching.

Do you believe that? God is perfect, and a perfect being cannot lie. Having the faith that God penned the Bible gives us the hope that what He says in it is true. God keeps his promises, and if your faith is in what He writes in the scriptures, then you can count on Him to be your comforter during labor and delivery.

The author of Galatians said that it was by faith that we receive the Comforter. What if we don't have that faith? What if our last birth was so traumatic that it would seem that any faith that was possible was snuffed out somewhere there in the delivery room? The scriptures declare that God is faithful, even when we are faithless (2 Timothy 3:13). It also says that faith comes by hearing, and hearing by the Word of God. That means that we get faith by hearing the scriptures.

Let me encourage you to fill your birth bag not only with slippers, socks, tennis balls, oils, etc., but mostly with scriptures that will be useful and encouraging to you. They will help you overcome Satan's fear and obtain the faith necessary to reap the benefits of our dear and wonderful Comforter!

Bible Study Discussion

1. What are your favorite Bible verses?

2. What other verses have you collected that encourage you in your pregnancy, labor and delivery?

3. How do you think the Bible will help you to have an easier birth?

4. What issues are you dealing with right now?

5. What part of this chapter stands out to you?

In Their Own Words

Birth Testimony # 1

From the Philippeans

We woke up a little before 6am on the 13th of November and Mary noted some contractions. There was absolutely no pain. When we timed them though, they came quite regularly every 5 minutes. We decided to go together to New Manila so Mary could have a check up perhaps in the afternoon at St Luke's Medical Center which is very near my office. (Our house is quite far from the hospital.) We prayed the prayer of Onset of Labor and called our spiritual elders in community who prayed over us and the baby in case this was the real thing.

Then we went about our morning prayers, routines and preparations. By 8:30am however, Mary noted an acceleration of the contractions and a bit of discomfort but the latter would dissipate as soon as she did the relaxed abdominal breathing and said some praises to the Lord. On the way to my office we timed the contractions again and noted them to be coming regularly at 2-3 minutes so we decided I would drop Mary off first at the hospital before proceeding to my meeting at the office.

When we got to the hospital room the resident wanted to do a non-stress test first thinking either Mary wasn't in labor yet or at least very early because she looked very comfortable. At her request however (they had to listen to her, she was an OB there!) the doctor conceded to check her first. To everyone's delight the resident reported she was already 6-7cm dilated! (You should have seen the look on her face as she was counting rom 1 to 7 during the checkup!)

I proceeded to read the prayers and meditations from Christ Centered Childbirth. Mary tried to concentrate on breathing correctly and repeating the meditations or agreeing with the prayers I would utter. We would also pray in tongues alternatively. As the contractions became more intense and more frequent Mary would note some pain coming but this would dissipate as we uttered prayers together.

A little before 12 noon we transferred to the Delivery Room (she was 10cm and fully dilated) and were instructed to push during the contractions. Mary tried to do so with all her might while I and the obstetrician who is also a Christian cheered her on. All throughout, we kept thanking the Lord that each contraction, overwhelming though it seemed, would just have to be ridden with, and was bringing us closer to the birth of our beloved baby. After 2 hours of 2nd stage labor however, our baby had not yet been delivered. (It was confirmed later on that the baby was simply too big, especially for an Asian woman!) Jane remembered what you wrote that if there was something the doctor needed to do to help medically, we needed to trust that the Lord may want to use this. Mary asked her obstetrician if the baby was in position for assisted vaginal delivery with vacuum extraction and her OB agreed that everything was just right for this. (Otherwise, they might have considered doing a CS because it was already 2 hrs) At 2:48pm our baby Mark was born into this world weighing 3.670 kgs, with an apgar score of 9 / 9, very healthy and such a beautiful child!

Our obstetrician was so ministered by the process of Christ-centered childbirth. She wants to get to know more about it too. The Lord is truly faithful and every good and perfect gift comes from Him!

Jesus be praised!

Birth Testimony # 2

It was my daughter's fourth child, but first experience with a doula, and my first experience with a military hospital. The room was very small and white everywhere. It reminded me of an emergency room. You know, the tiny rooms you go crazy in waiting and waiting for the doctor to come in and see you? She was not yet in labor, but had been battling with gestational diabetes and hypertension throughout her pregnancy. The doctors were eager to deliver as soon as possible.

There was a problem, and they looked concerned when they did the ultrasound. The baby was in a side-lying position, called "transverse." They calmly told my daughter that her baby would have to be delivered via c-section, unless she wanted to let them try a "version." That is a procedure where the doctors attempt to manually turn the baby to a head-down position by manipulating it from the outside of the mother's stomach. This can be a very painful process and also carries some risk. She and her husband asked the doctors to let us talk about it and when they left the room we joined hands and prayed. Steve boldly asked the Lord to turn that baby to a head down position so that she could not only deliver vaginally, but to spare her from having to have the version done.

When the doctors returned to the room, they informed them that they were willing to try the version. Because of the risks involved, the version had to be performed in the surgical suite, so we would have to wait until after lunch so that they had time to get everyone in place for the procedure.

Finally we were led to the surgical suite and my son-in-law and I were robed and masked so that we could go in and be with her. I stood by her head stroking her hair as they got the ultra sound machine ready to find the baby's exact position. I looked around the room and there were about 10 students in there to witness the procedure, along with the surgical team and my son-in-law and I. It was quite crowded, so I stayed by her head so that she could focus on me, and her husband held her hand and continued to pray...

When they had the ultrasound machine in place and began the scan, the doctor got a confused look on her face. Then looked a few seconds more before announcing that the baby had indeed moved to a head-down position on his own!! Now THAT was a God thing! The students filed out of the room one by one, obviously disappointed that they were not going to learn about a version that day. But, we were rejoicing and giving God all of the glory!

About 4 hours later my grandson was born in an un-medicated, vaginal birth, completely healthy at 8 pounds 13 ounces. We all cried and everyone there knew they had witnessed the hand of God that day! It did not matter that the room was not decorated with frills and homey looking furniture. Nor did it matter that the military staff was pretty much 30 years behind in the idea of a "natural" birth. GOD was there and that made it one of the best births I have ever attended.

Birth Testimony # 3

This last pregnancy I had Braxton Hick's like contractions in the last week of my pregnancy. I was achy and restless and gasy and had loose stools too. On my last day of pregnancy there was a slow shift in the way my contractions felt to me: The braxton Hicks like contractions involved my whole abdomen. My back was already sore so I couldn't use the front vs. back to front differentiation. My contractions went from feeling like my whole belly was getting hard (for a long and indefinite time and at very irregular intervals) to deep set pains in my low abdomen and then to definite cramp like feelings in my groin and cervix...I knew it was my cervix because I remembered what it felt like when the baby had been kicking me there previously.

The night I went into unmistakable labor was a school night for me. I had gone to my husband's office downtown in Chicago with our other three children and was to drop them off at 6, go to class until 9 and then ride the train home (a 30-45 minute trip) and get there around 10 PM. I had felt like I needed to urinate all day without any real results and I had been kind of crampy and sore all week along with loose stools on and off so I wasn't sure with my head that I was so close. But my heart and spirit knew. Even though I wasn't sure, I asked my husband to hang around with the kids at a nearby park or at his office until my class was over. My mind wasn't convinced that this was it, but my spirit kept telling me that I would regret having to take the train home if my heart bent to fear and doubt and chose to let Louis go back home without me.

So, during class, the transition I talked about above began. The contractions were still irregular and seemed a half hour or more apart (though I was trying to be a good student and pay attention to the teacher and not so much the clock, so I can't be sure) and so I thought, well maybe I need to go to the bathroom. I'd been having pretty serious pressure sensations for about two weeks. I figured the Drs. were just right that my baby was "REALLY well" engaged and that it still wasn't time. I was just close. My due date was the 7th and it was the 3rd of September, so it would make sense for me to "feel" close, right? If only I had paid attention to my feelings earlier. I could have been home relaxing instead of in a cramped position on an art bench wondering...should I stay or should I go?

Class was over at 9:00 but I was pretty sure at 8:30 that this wasn't just "false labor". I'm not sure that there really is such a thing anymore actually. I think it should all be considered early labor. Maybe we could look at it more positively then. Our bodies getting an early start and getting us to the big day gradually instead of in a rush. Anyway, when class ended I picked up all my gear and headed back to my husband's office down the street. I met him and the kids on the sidewalk on the way, and asked him to get them back in the car while I went in to go to the bathroom again and call my mom "just in case".

You should have seen the look on his face when I told him I wasn't sure if I was in labour. "I think so..." I said "but I can't really tell.." I think that it was just so fast and different than the three times before. By now it seemed the contractions were a great deal more uncomfortable (I was really waddling around...I felt like I was walking around my baby's head!) and about five minutes or so apart. But I didn't have a watch on and couldn't really count. They still didn't seem very long or hard to bear, though.

Anyway, he went to the car with the kids and I went inside. I was recalling at this point, as I headed for the bathroom one more time (obeying the pressure I felt as my baby moved down further into my pelvis), the story Jenn had told me about her "accidental homebirth"...not so much pain as she expected (memories of pitocin). Felt like she had to pee really bad. I had told my husband the week before that as soon as my cervix opens this baby is going to just fall right out of me. So I'm thinking...what if this baby is crowning? Oh God, help me be strong and ready for your will in this birth!

Went to the bathroom. No relief. No results. But no crowning either!!! :) So I still had time and unfortunately still some doubt. I called my mom and told her to get the car and dad ready in case this was it. I would try to time my contractions a little better in the car and call her when I got home if I was sure this was it.

In the car the contractions were getting closer and closer, five to three minutes apart then, but the intensity wasn't a lot greater or the length of each one either. Here...still doubt. Plus I was having a lot of trouble concentrating on the math of it all, and wasn't real sure of the time that had lapsed between contractions. Now I was praying the whole time, too. What is this Lord? Make me sure. Help me to work with my body and make the right decisions and wait for the right time to call the doctor and hospital and family. I think this is another hang up us women have. Thinking that our labours have to follow the text book to be "real" labour. Thinking this way had given the enemy room to keep me in doubt. My mind was ruling my heart and my heart my spirit. I still hadn't given in and given up to the real Ruler of my spirit in this very important matter. And my anxious doubt was working on becoming fear.

We got home and I called my mom and told her I thought they should come and apologized for not being really sure, but wanted her to be here if this was really it. I warned her that if this was it, then she might not make it in time to be there for the labour. I apologized for that too.

Then I tried to call my brother, who would have to be at my house before I left for the hospital in order for my husband to be with me the whole time. I left a message with him that I would call him back in a half hour. I had to pack a bag!!!...remember I thought for sure I would go "late" in my pregnancy again? I was worried about talking to my doctors about how long they would let me go without inducing. ....guess it wasn't so necessary. But the mind set had kept me from being as ready as I could have been. I hadn't finished my verses book. I hadn't copied support notes for my dear husband into his reminders flipbook yet. I hadn't gone over anything with him again besides our original sharing of ideas and suggestions. I hadn't checked my e-mail for scripture Julie had sent. I could have at least read it. But God had another lesson He thought was more important than a memory verse or two, as helpful as those are.

A half an hour went by and the contractions were defintely five minutes or less apart by now. My mind was clearing a bit and I had my watch on now and my bag packed (mostly) and I was able to concentrate enough to write down the time each time the peak hit. I was never good at telling when the contraction really was starting...only when it was full on. I figure one peak to another was probably as reliable at least as one start to another. Finally!!! My mind was switching from what should be happening and what I should be doing to what I needed to do and figuring out my own way to labour.

I'm praying through each contraction...talking really...to God. Before labour started this time, I never thought I would be able to be calm enough in spirit to do this, but there I was doing it any how. I'm claiming the promises we have all been talking about from His Word. Reminding Him (myself really) of His faithfulness. Asking Him to keep me faithful to His plan for this birth and to my love for this baby. Please don't let me crumble and give in to fear and pain. Be my strength through this contraction and the next. This is a battle of my flesh and the enemy against the spirit you have given me in Christ. Silence the "old man" you nailed to the cross for me. Bind her up and keep her from me. Strengthen the "new man" in me to speak in your truth and love and Spirit against her. Give me your wisdom and strength and courage. Help me to stay true to this child and to you and to my family as a witness and child myself as this labour progresses to transition. I admit my fear to you of that time. I remember still the pain of my last three transitions and the desperation I felt then....Help me Lord! Help me, please...

Okay. Now I call the hospital. No answer at the doctor's office like there was my previous labour (silly me, I had never asked the doctor who I should call this time), giving me the on call number for that evening. The voice inside telling me that I could still be wrong and should talk to the doctor first and do all these other things first before calling the hospital was scolded into silence every time it spoke up. AMEN!!! The LORD was answering my prayers. I dialed and told them I was in labour 2-3 minutes apart and was coming in. Astonished at the force and sureness in my voice the nurse said, "...um uh okay...".

I called my brother and got him finally, but he was too far away to get to our home soon. So I went to the living room and awoke my exhausted husband who was napping "just in case" in the middle of a mass of also slumbering little bodies. "It's time." I said, "I'm sure now and we can't wait any longer for Pat or mom and dad. We'll have to go now and Pat (my brother)will meet us there as soon as he can." He was astonished at the change in my voice too and stumbled around a bit as he took the bag I had packed and our three kids down to the car while I made some last minute calls to bring Louis' mom down from Wisconsin and Louis' best friend to the north side from the south side of Chicago for his big event.

I was pretty sure now that no one else would make it, but strangely I wasn't worried about it any more. As that "old man" tried to fill my head with what ifs...God's Spirit in me reminded me that He is sufficient. In Him is the fulness of the Godhead bodily. In Him I am complete. He will gently lead them that HAVE (taking this as having right now, in birth) young. He is with me always. He will carry me through this. He died for me. He rose for me. He is faithful, even when I believe not, because He can not deny Himself. This is His operation in me. Those who fear the Lord are blessed. He is their help and their shield. We got in the car and were on the way.

We were rushing, though the hospital was only five minutes away, because I knew and told my husband it wouldn't be long now. This was going to be fast. But I wasn't scared. I was thanking God (even now!!! Even as the intensity of the contractions finally started to grow) that He had sent me to all of you...that He had given me so much knowledge to renew my mind...and support and encouragement to refresh my heart...and such an abundance of truth and love and wisdom to strengthen my spirit.

I got to the hospital and had to check in at emergency myself while my husband parked the car and brought our boys in and waited for my brother to arrive and take over watch of them. I was admitted, went to the labor/delivery floor and suite all "alone". I was surprised at the presence of mind and confidence I still had to request all I had laid out previously in my labor plan. They had already gotten me into my "gown" and started to set up the room as I told them I wanted the labouring pool (tub) and they had to switch me to another room. Before I would have felt badly, but just followed them matter of factly while they exchanged glances and shrugged, and smilingly obligded.

Once there, I got a hep lock for my antibiotics and they started the first round. I got hooked up for the initial hour long fetal and mother monitoring. All my vitals were checked and I went through the manditory Q and A with one nurse as my doctor came in to check where we were in labour. A full 5 cm and at 0 station. Another prayer answered!!! I was definitely in active labour, though the edge of the contractions was bearable and my mood was light and cheery between peaks. I was as surprised as the nurses at this attitude and the doctor and nurses were all surprised that I was so far along already and that I was still so good humored despite the intensity of the contractions they were reading on the monitor.The doctor nodded at the nurses with a shrug and a smile (a lot of that going on) and they all commented that they didn't think it would be long and that I may not get both doses of antibiotics or to use the tub tonight. I had arrived in the room at 11:35 PM and by about 12:10 or so my contractions had gotten to 1 and a 1/2 to 2 min apart.

Somehow my focal point became the clock on the wall with the second hand by then. Still I wasn't worried. Still there was this peace. I just knew inside that it may be even shorter than the nurses and doctor expected. I couldn't get comfortable physically. I felt restless but didn't feel like I could get my body to move out of the position I was in. I was getting pretty sure that I wouldn't make it through the first hour of monitoring to when they would change me over to the ambulatory monitor I would use in the tub. I was very sure that they would never get the tub filled by the time I would be pushing. It was a big tub!!! Nothing would go exactly as planned that night. I knew it. My heart resounded with my spirit though. AMEN!!! It's okay!!! He is sufficient!!! It felt so good to trust in my Lord!!!

Well, around the time they were switching me over to the ambulatory monitor and offering me a birthing ball or a trip to the bathroom (they could see my restlessness and hear my moans of discomfort by now) my husband finally came in. Oh to see his face!!! And it was confident though questioning with the same intensity of excitement as I was feeling now. I filled him in on where we were and he sat beside me and held my hand and smiled at me lovingly. He's not much of a talker but I could see the Lord working in his heart as I had asked in prayer so fervently. He was there with me and was confident and hopeful and ready. Oh God. Thank you!!! I don't think I stopped singing that out all night ...right along with help me, help me, help me's at the peaks of contractions which were pretty intense by now.

About the contractions. They were intense only at the peak. It was that the urge to bear down was already strong. It hurt to resist.

172

There was so much pressure and the peaks were piggy backing. I was begging God aloud through each urge to help me and be my strength and silently to stop my body from pushing until the time was right, protect my body and baby, and help us progress and thrive in this together. I was also able to talk with my dear husband this time. Though I think the time between contractions was shorter than with the other births they seemed longer. It was almost like time and thought about everything else were stilled in those moments. I just looked at my husband and murmered requests for touch and hugs and snuggles and words. Not ashamed. Not feeling as though I asked too much of him or anyone else. I was absorbed in our togetherness and in the Lord's presence there and in the anticipation of SUCH an event!!! God is so good, God IS. Period.

The nurses thought I was talking to them when I was talking to God...screaming at one point...but it didn't really hurt to do that either. I just felt a huge release as I gave up my weakness and labour to Him. I realized around this time (slow learner that I am) that He just wanted me to trust in Him alone. He would provide the support and technical help and time and place and experience and strength for me. I just had to let go, and let it happen.

The nurses around me couldn't answer my cries. My husband was with me but in the midst of it all just like me wrapped up in me...my one flesh...he is precious! But only God is sufficient to be all I need and desire in one Body and Spirit!!! He is the LIVING God!!!

I still hit a wall in this waiting. I asked the nurse to check me because I was sure I was so close to having this baby. I felt desperate to bear down!!! I thought it was hard to deal with before on pain meds....but the intensity of my body's push toward delivery was astounding! (Don't ever let anyone tell you your body is not able to do the work it was designed to do.) So I was at 9 cm at the peak of contractions now 12:50 or so I'm guessing....I had forgotten the clock by now, you'll imagine, but there was a lip on my cervix at both sides. No pushing yet. Ugh. She suggested they break my waters so that I would get to full dilation and pushing faster. I was at the wall like I told you. The enemy took another opportunity and I submitted to the idea. But God was in control and it never happened.

The intensity of fighting and straining against the urge to push was taking its toll on my already sore and tired (from the last weeks of pregnancy) back and I asked to be helped into another position. They got me on my left side, informing me that it was too far along now to get me up, though I wanted to stand. I think they were sure that I wouldn't be able to resist pushing or that gravity would do the job too quickly if I did.

I was checked again at my asking by a resident who was assisting on the floor that night and then by my doctor to decide if she agreed that it would be okay for me to start pushing now. I still had a bit of a lip, but she thought that she could ease it around the baby if we were careful in pushing. I was so relieved that I would be allowed to push finally that I had no second thoughts.

As soon as the next urge hit its highest intensity, I beared down as the doctor supported my leg and my husband lovingly applied counterpressure to my hips and low back. The love in his eyes! I felt so surrounded by love and comfort and so supported! I can't remember seeing anything around me at this point...in the seconds of this contraction...the one contraction...the room spun and froze at the same time and all I could do was feel. My heart and my mind and my spirit were all focused and present and for an instant, I felt what it was like to be let go of by the flesh and to worship fully in spirit,feeling its reality. Then I felt the rush of a little life in a little body sweep out of me in two stages...one push put baby up to the shoulders into this world and then a second brought out the rest. The doctor shook her head in amazement and muttered her awe at the ease of the delivery, even when it went so quickly. There had to be trauma...somewhere...But the baby was healthy and pink and crying loudly! I was so anxious and eager to meet this little child. Praising/thanking God loudly in my heart and soul! But then, when I saw this baby the first time...O GOD!!!...a girl! It's a girl!!! My heart burst and I yelled it out to all the floor and to all the world!!! All the joy and thanksgiving and peace and hope flooded out of me in relief and happiness and glow and energy. Who knew it could be like this and who knew I would be so rewarded in His work?

I was awake and alert through it all. No interventions. I didn't even get my second round of antibiotics. I didn't get premature rupture of Membranes (PROM). The doctor went away with incredulity written all over her face...smiling from ear to ear...there was no damage to my cervix, vagina, uterus or perinium. The placenta was intact. The baby was healthy. Blood work later revealed that her blood was free of infection. And she was so beautifully shaped and with such clear skin because of the quick delivery. No trauma anywhere, though all searched for it and were surprised by the lack of it. The nurses walked away surprised at my alertness...saying I didn't even look like I had just had a baby...and they were glad to have had the chance to attend a nonmedicated birth, which they said were few and far between in their experience.

God is so good!!! Was it Julie who said that we had the promise of a safe and healthy delivery? That the baby and mother would be guarded? Such good news and so true that the Lord has hope and an expected end for us in all things!!!

HE IS FAITHFUL!!! HE IS MERCIFUL!!! HE IS GRACEFUL!!! He was with me fully. He delivered me from my fears and the hand of the enemy. He gave me not only what I needed through out but what we all desperately wanted. A little girl!!!

And now my boys can know how He answers prayers too! James and Bryan and Josh now have a little sister. Born at 1:10AM at 7 lbs. and 7 oz. the nurses called her "lucky" but I let them know she's blessed! We all are. At 20inches long, they called her strong and healthy, but I let them know she is cared for and loved! We all are.

Little Faith Anne's birth has taught me the lesson of her name. I don't believe I could ever falter in my faith in Christ again. He IS sufficient. But I KNOW, I have experienced, that even if I do waver in my belief, HE ABIDETH FAITHFUL. He can do all things. (I'm talking to those mothers-to-be that have posted recently and any others who will benefit from hearing it...)

When you hit a wall of fear and doubt during your labor (I did all three times) and you feel like you can't do it. You are right. And it's okay! HE does it. He does it all. He will deliver the child from your womb. It is He that does a good work in you, and through you, and for you and to His glory. Trust in Him and you will not be ashamed. AMEN!!! GOD is GOOD!!! and He is more than able to do exceedingly abundantly above. He delivered me right along with my little baby girl! He will deliver you too if you put your life, and your child's life, in His hands.

To my sisters...may He bless you with His awesome presence and peace and love and truth. May He give you knowledge and the understanding to impart it wisely. May He renew your minds and spirits with His Truth and Grace and Mercy daily. May He keep you and yours and enrich you and your ministries for Him greatly.

Birth Testimony # 4

I started contracting Thursday evening July 14th. It was consistent but stopped, started, stopped, etc. Not really painful but uncomfortable. Nothing progressed so I blew it off as pre-labor. Two days previous I had an OB check-up and was 4 cm.

Things around me were getting so stressful and out of control. I was crying a lot and felt like a basket case. Saturday I contracted most of the day but no progression in the pain or strength. I called a friend to get a few things off my chest and while talking to her she said "You have had 3 contractions during this 13 min conversation and you breathe harder and more concentrated with each one, you sure you're not in labor? I kind of stopped and observed the last few hours and thought... hmm... possibly.

I had nothing else to do so I decided I'd go get checked to see if I'd progressed. Since I tested positive for GBS I wanted to get there a decent time, at least this way I'd have an idea, but to be honest I really didn't think I was in labor, but hoped I was. I was checked to be a stretch 4 cm. The nurse wanted me to walk for an hour and she would check me to see if there was a change and we'd go from there, because I was contracting every 5 - 6 min. Therefore, we walked (my sister and husband). My husband stopped at a restroom in the hall way and I continued on to my room to use the restroom.

I heard this pop sound and a splash,,,, stood up and nothing was running out of me so I thought "maybe my water broke but I'm not sure" I told my sister I was suspicious that my water may have broke, but the fact that I was not leaking made me question it. She noted the time and we walked on. About 3 min later a contraction hit me and it was like night and day difference, I knew then that my water had broke. I wanted to keep walking but it was only 3 more min later that another contraction came so we headed back toward my room. I had my sister call my Doula and she was on the way. Took me three contractions to get back and each one dropped me to my knees and the birthing song began.

My nurse saw me on my knees in the hall and said "well that's a big difference, lets check you" (my husband was still in the bathroom and my 2 year old was holding my hand saying "Sorry Mamma." I kept kissing him and smiling and talking so he wouldn't panic. My husband came in the room, not knowing a darn thing was happening and I told him to call the sitter, he said "Shouldn't we wait till she checks you and see if you changed?" I had another contraction and could tell by the look on his face he was caught of guard and confused.

He called the sitter while I was checked and found to be 6/7 cm. (this was after about 30 min of walking). The nurse started getting things ready and called some more nurses for help because I was going so fast. But I was having a great time laughing in between. About 4 contractions after being checked I told the nurse that I thought I was feeling pushy. She did a quick check (she was great checking me in what ever position I was in) and I was complete, she told me to go ahead and do what ever my body wanted.

My doula arrived just before then. My husband left the room with our son who was getting a bit worried. I put the bottom of the bed down and got my knees and panted, breathed and pushed a little through the peek. The whole time I was so aware of everything around me and enjoyed every moment of it, I could feel my son moving down through my pelvis and was aware of what was happening.

It was great. My Doula was talking to me and reminding me of all the things I told her I wanted to hear (Thank you Heather) and my sister was loving on me (Twin sister) and backing up what my Doula said. The resident DR came in while we waited for my DR. She wasn't so great, asked me several times to get in a sitting position and I refused, my sister finely told her to stop asking and told her I was happy and content on my knees.

At that point she also kept saying "lets wait for the Doctor, stop pushing and wait, I told her that she better get ready because I was having this baby with or without a DR. The second my DR walked in she said "I need you to roll over and get in a sitting position now." I heard my DR say "no, she can stay just like that and have her baby however she wants to. I'm here Sara, you're doing great, keep it up" I laughed and said "Hey, typical Dr Hardin, you show up just In time to catch my baby" We all laughed because my last birth went fast (not this fast) and he barely made it for the catch. So my baby crowned and head was born, but..........

Shoulders were stuck, I delivered one shoulder but the other wouldn't come out, I heard my doctor say to the resident doctor, "You gonna get that baby out now? If not, move out of my way" She didn't respond so he said "move" and he told my husband, "I need her on her back now" I could hear a little panic in the room and I was flipped over like a pancake in a skillet. I even laughed out loud because I was blown away at the strength of my husband and doula and sister to flip me like

177

that. They lifted my legs, one more push and my baby was out, however, his body was very pink and face and head total blue.

The DR put him on me and the nurses started rubbing him, I knew things weren't right and everyone was saying its ok, but we knew better. I started roughing him up and talking to him trying to get a response. They cut his cord and took him off to the side, where I noticed about 5 nurses around him. Everyone was very nice about moving all the stuff so I could see them working on my son. But I still couldn't see everything. My sister went to his side making me feel much better and my husband kind of backed away, a bit panicked. Later she told me they performed some CPR on him and put a tube in his lungs to suck out all the fluid. Seemed like forever, but it was only about 2 or 3 min and he was breathing and turning pink.

The other members of my birthing team got to the hospital but when they got there, things were too hectic and busy to let anyone in. From my water breaking (and any pain starting) and birth, it was 58 Min. Praise GOD!! It was short. I felt so satisfied right away and just can't believe what an amazing experience I had. My doula commented on how amazing my sister and I worked together like we were one person. I can't say or express what a great experience it was.

Birth Testimony # 5

My first two births were completely natural hospital births, with no disruption. I had taken Bradely classes and was very committed to birthing without medication or intervention. I was thirsty for knowledge and truth in an area that I was totally unfamiliar with. The book, "Childbirth Without Fear" was a pillar in my birth knowledge, and perhaps was all I really needed to get through birth at the time. My walk with the Lord was new and I really didn't include Him much in the process.

The first was a very typical 24 hour start-to-finish labor, done without the help of a doula, and husband asleep on the chair through the night. I was my own coach for the most part, and during second stage my husband was a champion advocate. No one asked me if I wanted medication, there was no IV, and the monitor was used rarely. If I could change anything about that birth, I would not allow them to take my baby from me immediately after birth, so that I could bond better with her. I regret that to this day. Other than that, it was an amazing experience that reshaped my entire life.

My second was an amazing birth, with my daughter being in the posterior position for the entire process. She was born face up, looking right at God from the beginning. The pain of a posterior labor is forever etched on my mind, yet I wouldn't change a thing about it, because the joy that followed the trial was magnified beyond belief. It is almost embarrassing to watch the video, because I carried on for about ten minutes, whooping and laughing, crying songs of love to my new baby. I think the hard work really revved me up for extraordinary joy.

The first thing I thought of when I saw the second line in the pregnancy window of my third child was, "Oh no, I have to go through labor again." I stuffed that thougth away and told myself that it would be just fine, no worries. About half-way through my pregnancy, someone recommended the book Supernatural Childbirth to me. I read it, and was amazed at the concept of a painless birth. I was a little concerned about the use of scripture being declared to mean something out of context, but I could not deny her testimonies. I worried that if I had a painful birth, I might feel like I didn't have enough faith, but I knew that somehow, right or wrong, God honored her faith.

I decided that I was going to begin to pray for the same things she had been praying for. Still, there was doubt in my mind that it was possible for me, since my last birth was so long and difficult. I asked God to show me exactly how it would be possible, and sure enough, He did.

One afternoon I was lying on my bed with my daughter, taking a nap, when I felt someone take their fingers and gather the skin up on my forehead. It startled me and I opened my eyes to see who had done it, but no one was there. I prayed and asked God what was happening, and I felt in my spirit that God wanted to show me something.

Shortly thereafter, my two year old daughter sat up in her sleep, adjusted her position, and then threw herself backwards and landed her hard head right on my forehead. It sounded like the perverbial watermelon dropped on cement, and my husband who had just walked in rushed over to see if I was allright.

The funny thing was, I didn't feel a thing. I reassured my husband, and went back to resting.

"What was that for, God?" I asked.

"When your daughter slammed her head into yours, I had my hand over your forehead. That is the hand you felt earlier pinching your skin. I am going to do the same thing to your cervix."

I truly felt in my heart that the Lord was saying this to me. I rushed to my friends at church that night, and they looked at me like I

179

was crazy. One of them was worried that I would feel like a failure during birth when it hurt, because the book Supernatural Childbirth was setting me up for dissappointment. I realized that I had to pray about this on my own, and not seek any support for a painless birth from others. I kept it secret, between me and my husband, because my friend had gone to one of the pastors with the issue, concerned for my spirit. The pastor told them that painless birth wasn't scriptural, and that we should come in and talk to him. We didn't.

At seven months, I thought my water had broken, so I went in for litmus strip testing and a half-hour on the external fetal monitor. When they put that on me and left the room, I developed an anxiety attack that could kill a horse, because it caused me to recall my second labor. I had known for eight years that fear would produce more pain, yet I couldn't get over my own. I asked God, no pleaded with Him, to help me overcome the fear.

While driving through town a few days later, I passed an auto repair shop that had a marquee which usually had scripture on it. By the time I saw it, I only had time to read 1 John 4:18. I went home and looked it up, and it was in fact a scriputure God had put there for me. It talked about how perfect love would cast out fear. I knew the only one who had perfect love was God, so I began to trust Him that He would take away the fear when the time came. I worried all the way up to my day of delivery, you know.

I had been having false labor for about three weeks, and it was two weeks before my due date, so I figured that this was just some more of the same. I decided to take my daughters and the neighbor girl to the café and Walmart for a girls night out. Usually we would be having a great time, but for some reason, they were really getting on my nerves! While in Walmart, I had to lean on the basket during contractions, but they weren't bad at all. I was just so tired. Tired of being pregnant.

I was tired of people aksing me when my due date was. Every time I went to the market, they would make wise cracks about how big I was, like a basket ball in the front. This didn't bother me as much, because I had heard that boys were supposed to be all in front, and we really wanted a boy. I refused to get an ultrasound because Grantly Dick-Read M.D. had said that when the mothers were full of joy, they did not hemorrhage, but those who were not happy tended to bleed more. I remembered the joy when finding out the gender, and how that joy wipes away all memory of the trials. I knew that it was an important aspect of birth, and I didn't want to cheat and find out early.

No, the basket ball remarks were actually welcome. It was the large comments that bothered me. By the end of my pregnancy in December, when people would ask me when my due date was, I would tell them April 1st. The look on their faces was priceless and few got the joke.

We left Walmart and went home happy. My husband had a long day at work and was also tired. We went to bed around ten o'clock, and about fifteen minutes after falling asleep, I felt a pop and a warm gush on my leg. Honey….. He wasn't too impressed. "Are you sure…" he asked. Yes, dear….

I think the thing I was worried about most was having the baby on the freeway, since we lived over an hour away from the hospital. Well, the hospital we chose to deliver at. We drove right past the hospital with the NICU because they were notorious for taking the baby away from you right after birth and leaving them in the nursery for unnecessary and almost rediculous reasons.

I was worried about the long drive, and the bumps along the way. The funny thing was, by the time we got to the hospital, I didn't want to get out, I was so comfortable. The heater was warm, the music was soothing, and my husband was in charge. I had worried the whole pregnancy, but when the time came, God indeed took away all fear. Even on the long drive there.

We went in, and my friend arrived to watch the kids. I told the nurse that I didn't really want her to check me because I was afraid that I would only be at 2 cm, and therefore didn't want to know. At four o'clock, she asked if she could check me since I had been laboring for three hours at the hospital.

I was in the rocking chair, and I needed her help to get up, so she wrapped her arms around me to pull me up. My husband had been doing a marvelous and sufficient job at coaching, but there was something so soothing about her arms, like a mother's arms, that I didn't want to let go of her.

She checked me and got a funny look on her face. She said my cervix was too far back to reach, so she couldn't tell how dilated it was. Later, my friend said that she came into the room and told them that I was only at two centimeters. Good thing she didn't tell me…

My contractions did not hurt at all, but I could feel pressure in my back. I knew he was posterior. I was very tired from all the walking in Walmart and thought if I could only get down in a squat somehow, but how? I think the nurse must have read my mind, and suggested the birth ball. I sat down on it and leaned on some pillows we had stacked up.

I changed my prayer a little and added a part where I gave my body permission to open up and let the baby out. I soon felt my baby flip into the right position. My husband sat behind me and held a warm compress to my back. About forty-five minutes later, I looked back at him and saw that he didn't have his hand on the warm compress anymore. Before I could ask him to put his hand back, another contraction came and it was full of pain and I let out a moan much like the one I used when birthing my second child. Hmmm, I thought. Guess it is going to get bad now. He put his had back, and I returned to greeting contractions with my prescribed prayer. I didn't realize how important having his hand on my back was.

About ten minutes later, the contractions stopped. I think fifteen minutes must have gone by, so I figured it would be a good time to go to the toilet. Since the contractions didn't hurt, I assumed I was still in early labor. They only hurt that one time when my focus was distracted and my routine was interrupted.

While on the toilet, I got that all-too-familiar urge to push. The nurse came in and checked me, and I was at eight centimeters. No, I couldn't push yet, she said. She went to call the doctor in and I was hit with another heavy contraction. I couldn't help but to push, and I felt my cervix burning. Geesh, I told myself. You just ripped your cervix!

It was the most powerful thing I had ever felt in my life. I was standing there by the bed, and the contractions were coming right on top of each other. I wondered if the head was getting close, so I checked. He was about an inch from the opening, so I yelled for my husband to call the nurse. Before she could come in, I delivered his head. When she arrived, she asked if I could give one good push. Unfortunately, my efforts were in vain, because his little shoulder was stuck on my pubic bone.

She asked me to get on the bed, but I was frozen. I literally couldn't move. They both took an arm and lifted me up on the side of the bed, and she pushed on my pubic bone to dislodge the shoulder. He was purple, but breathing and crying. She said that she might take him to the hall for some oxygen, but I said twice, "Please don't take my baby." She reluctantly agreed and gave him oxygen at the bedside, and he recovered quickly.

From the time she checked me at two centimeters, to the time he was born, was one hour. Only twice during that time did I feel any pain. Once while I awoke out of a dreamy state to see my husband resting and was alert and disrupted, and the other time when my cervix stretched. The rest of the contractions were painless and it did not hurt when he was coming out. Perhaps because it was my third, maybe it was because I was standing, I don't know. A friend of mine once asked me if it "*really* didn't hurt." I explained to her that although the vast majority didn't hurt, it did feel like pressure and it was a lot of work to stay relaxed and calm. It wasn't effortless, but it by no means was painful at all. I remember one of the first things I thought of after the birth was that I couldn't wait to do it again. And no, I don't think painless birth is unscriptural. In fact, Galatians 3:13 says that we are redeemed from the curse of the law. The very first law, to not eat of the fruit, brought a discipline on women that did indeed cause painful birth. Be we do not live in the Old Testament. We have a God who has given us a new law, to love Him with all our heart and soul, and to love each other. There is no fear in that love, He is our comforter, and the fear of birth is abolished. We make choices out of the love for our child, and birth returns to normal. Do I believe that a painful birth is a sign of a lack of faith? Certainly not! I just do not, and will not believe that all women are pre-ordained to have a terrible time. Will my next birth be painless? Only God knows. I trust Him, though, to give me exactly the birth I need, so that I will learn the lesson that He has for me. Each of my births were different, and I learned priceless lessons with each of them. I wouldn't trade any of my birth stories. I had a typical birth, a birth that is considered one of the hardest ways of having a baby, and one without pain. I think the last birth was different, because I honored the Lord, having grown in my walk with Him. The nurses, knowing my history of long births, asked me what I did differently. I responded with one simple truth, "I prayed."

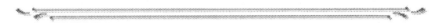

Bible Study Discussion

1. What positive birth stories can you share with the group?

2. Which birth story stood out to you?

3. Perhaps you might watch another positive birth video tonight.

4 Spend time in prayer together…

Chapter Fourteen
Medical Procedures

It is our responsibility as parents to seek out the information needed to make informed decisions. In a perfect world, the provider could educate you completely on all the pros and cons of the various potential interventions, but the truth is that they simply do not have the time. Childbirth education classes are a good place to begin, but many times are overcrowded and individual questions go unanswered due to lack of time. There is a wealth of information out there, thanks to the Internet, and parents are more equipped than ever to inform themselves. As a word of caution, make sure the source you are studying is reliable and not overly biased. The internet is full of anecdotal information and can be very unreliable. Look at both ends of the spectrum and make your own decisions.

The following are some procedures that you might need to make a decision about. Listed are the pros and cons of each procedure, and it is up to you to decide if it is something you would like to voluntarily take part in. In some instances, medical intervention may be necessary and you will have to trust your care provider. You have freedom of choice, and you will fare better if you have full knowledge of your alternatives.

Artificial Rupture Of Membranes (AROM)

The attendant uses a crochet-like hook to rupture the amniotic sack, in order to speed labor up, administer an internal fetal monitor, or prevent baby from being born in the bag of waters.

THE BENEFITS

~ May help speed labor
~ Allows caregiver to see the color of amniotic fluid to assess fetal distress
~ Allows caregiver to apply a fetal scalp electrode in the event that close fetal heart tone monitoring is indicated

THE PROBLEMS

~ Sets timeline for delivery
~ Most caregivers want mother to deliver within 24 hours (Increases your chances of labor augmentation or cesarean section)
~ Unwise to do prior to 4cm
~ Could cause cord prolapse, which is life-threatening to the baby
~ Breaks the germ barrier
~ Labor contractions are often more intense without the cushion of amniotic fluid

ALTERNATIVES

~ Avoid unnecessary induction, narcotics, and the epidural. Other natural methods of speeding labor include methods such as nipple stimulation, upright positions, hydration, mental acceptance of the process, relaxation, and avoiding fear-tension-pain. Another method is to help the baby to become better applied to the cervix by assuming positions that help. Squatting, lunging, hip rotations, stair climbing, abdominal lifting, resting in the jacuzzi, showering, and slow dancing are popular and effective ways to speed labor.

NOTE: Never rupture the membranes to induce labor. Labor can easily stall or stop if the cervix is not at 4cm yet. If you have not delivered 24 hours after rupture, many hospitals and physicians will require a cesarean. Rupturing the membranes before fully confident that active labor is underway can be risky.

Stripping the Membranes

The care provider loosens the lower segment of the amniotic sac from the cervix by running a finger around the inside part of the cervix. It is thought that this causes labor to begin sooner.

THE BENEFITS

~ Onset of labor may occur 4 days sooner
~ Good for women with gestational diabetes or large baby

THE PROBLEMS

~ A slight increase of cesarean sections
~ Does not reduce the number of inductions
~ Procedure is uncomfortable, causes cramping, bleeding, or spotting
~ Procedure is often done without the woman's knowing or permission.

Prostaglandin Gel

Prostaglandin gel contains the hormone prostaglandin that is used to soften the cervix, preparing it for dilation. The doses are administered directly to the cervix every four to eight hours

THE BENEFITS

~ May start contractions
~ Prepares cervix if Pitocin is needed

THE PROBLEMS

~ Contains pig or bull semen
~ Possible epileptic seizure
~ Possible tetanic contractions
~ Possible cervical Rupture
(Information may be found in package insert found at www.drugs.com/pdr/prepidil_gel.html)

Cervidel

Similar to prostaglandin, Cervidil is used for induction, placed on an applicator and inserted inside the vagina, with a string attachment allowing for removal.

Learn more about Cervidil at:
http://www.drugs.com/MMX/Dinoprostone.html

THE BENEFITS

~ Ability to remove medication on demand
~ May ripen the cervix and induce contractions

THE PROBLEMS

~ Anaphylaxis shock (allergy)
~ Bradycardia (slow heart beat)
~ Asthma-like symptoms
~ peripheral vasoconstriction (pale, cool, or blotchy skin on arms or legs; weak or absent pulse in arms or legs) —possibly severe
~ Chest pain or pressure
~ Tachycardia (Fast heart beat)
~ Severe cramping of the uterus
~ Diarrhea
~ Abdominal or stomach cramps
~ Fever (about 50% chance with 20 mg suppositories- may lead to c-sec
~ if membranes are ruptured)
~ Nausea/vomiting
~ Headache

ALTERNATIVES

~ Avoid unnecessary induction
~ Try natural labor induction techniques (ask a local midwife)

External Fetal Monitor

The monitor is a machine that records the baby's heart rate over time as well as the strength of the contractions. This is accomplished by placing two belts around the mother's abdomen. The belt at the top is for the contractions and the belt below is for the fetal heart rate.

Some hospitals require that the monitor continuously, others require that it is used once every hour or two, and a select few are willing to only require a positive reading when you are assessed, and then will monitor you with a hand-held Doppler.

The monitor is a machine rolled in on a cart, has cords that go from your side to the machine, and requires that you remain close to the unit, often times in the bed in order for it to detect the baby's heart. There are some hospitals that have a cordless unit that allows you to get up and move around. Ask your provider if this is available for monitoring if needed.

THE BENEFITS

~ Allows caregiver an overall picture of the labor pattern

~ Artificial rupture of membranes is not necessary

~ Frequency of contractions easily assessed

~ Allows caregiver to get an idea of how the baby is tolerating the contractions

> This can prevent a fetal emergency by alerting the caregiver to the need of immediate intervention. This can be as simple as changing positions, or as extreme as cesarean section

THE PROBLEMS

~ Restricts movement affecting optimal fetal positioning
    (Heart tones typically picked up when woman is on her BACK)

~ Reliable tracing difficult when
        - Woman is obese or active.
        - Baby moves or is active.
        - Machine picks up maternal heart tones.
~ Uncomfortable to wear
        - Anything that disrupts the mother's ability to relax initiates the fear-tension-pain cycle.

~ Acceptable degrees of variation in the fetal heart rate have never been firmly established. This can lead to unnecessary intervention.
(Chalmers 1978; Haverkamp and Orleans 1983)

~ Has a high false-positive rate
        - It shows that baby is in
          distress when baby is actually fine.
        - Does not improve fetal outcomes.
        - raises cesarean rate

ALTERNATIVES

~ Some care providers are willing to do intermittent monitoring. For example, the initial assessment will be for an hour or two, and then for fifteen minutes at the top of each hour.
~ A hand-held Doppler unit, like what was used at your prenatal appointment, can be used .
~ It may be possible to negotiate an informed consent form

Internal Fetal Monitor

When the baby's heart rate is questionable or needs to be monitored continuously due to an induction or other procedure, the internal monitor will often be used. It is a scalp electrode, in the shape of a thin coil, twisted into the baby's scalp and directly picks up the pulse.

THE BENEFITS

~ Accurately monitors the fetal heart tones
    This is very necessary when baby is in distress and needs close
    monitoring.

THE PROBLEMS

~ Requires ruptured membranes
~ Uncomfortable
~ Scalp laceration
~ May be accidentally applied to cervix
~ Although rare, may be applied to baby's face with face presentation
~ Confining to bed and close proximity
~ Increases a sense of sickness, with more cords coming out of vagina

ALTERNATIVES

~ Avoid unnecessary induction
~ Avoid epidural anesthesia
~ Ask care provider if it is absolutely necessary.
~ Ask care provider if there are any alternatives.

Intravenous Fluids (IV)

Administered to laboring women for the purpose of giving her medication, liquids, or calories.

THE BENEFITS

Allows for intake if mother is nauseated.
Keeps calories up if care provider wants an empty stomach.
Maintains and open vein.
 Veins often collapse when hemorrhaging.
 In an emergency, there is one less step in starting an IV.

THE PROBLEMS

~Cumbersome/gives an impression of illness
~Can dilute the natural hormones in the bloodstream and if glucose is used, can affect mom's and baby's blood sugar/insulin levels.
~ Painful
~ Hydration and calories can be accomplished by mouth in a normal labor (The purpose of an empty stomach was outdated when women began to have cesareans with an epidural)

WHEN YOU MIGHT NEED IT

~ An extra long labor
~ Mother cannot keep anything down by mouth
~ If she is to receive general anesthesia
~ A condition exists that requires immediate medical intervention
 To administer certain medications
 GBS positive requires IV antibiotics

Alternatives

~ Hydrate and get calories by mouth
~ Ask for a saline-lock as a compromise

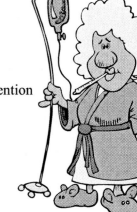

Pitocin

A synthetic form of oxytocin, the hormone needed to produce contractions. This is used either to start labor, speed up a slow labor, increase the strength of contractions, or stop a postpartum hemorrhage. It is primarily given by means of an intravenous fluid, yet can be given by injection.

THE BENEFITS

~ Can start or augment labor, when medically indicated
~ Can be turned off if necessary
~ Can be regulated and monitored closely
~ Can prevent or stop hemorrhage

THE PROBLEMS

~ Difficult to produce the natural progression of contractions
~ Pain from pitocin often more difficult to cope with
~ Requires an IV and constant fetal monitoring

From the manufacturers of Pitocin (insert)
- o maternal hypertensive episodes
- o cardiac arrhythmias
- o uterine spasm
- o titanic contraction
- o uterine rupture
- o subarachnoid hemorrhage
- o water intoxication
- o convulsions
- o coma
- o pelvic hemotoma
- o postpartum hemorrhage
- o afibrinogenemia
- o fetal death.

ALTERNATIVES

~ Avoid unnecessary induction
~ Avoid epidural anesthesia
~ Ask care provider if it is absolutely necessary.
~ Ask care provider if there are any alternatives.

Cytotec (misoprostol)

Cytotec is a small pill inserted into the birth canal and placed against the cervix, used to ripen the cervix and/or induce labor. The pill is usually broken in fourths, and one fourth is administered at a time.

THE BENEFITS

~ Cervical ripening agent
~ Able to induce or augment labor
~ Can stop postpartum hemorrhage
~ Allows person to go home after administrating the medication
~ Allows person to use the hot tub or shower
~ Does not require an IV
~ Quick labor

THE PROBLEMS

From the package insert located at:
http://www.pfizer.com/download/uspi_cytotec.pdf

~ Possible uterine rupture
~ Amniotic fluid embolism
   (Amniotic fluid gets into the blood stream)
~ Pelvic pain
~ Retained placenta
   (Placenta will not come out)
~ Severe vaginal bleeding
~ Shock
~ Fetal distress
~ Maternal and/or infant death
~ Long-term fetal effects unknown

~ Medication not evenly distributed throughout pill, possibility of getting all or none of medication in a divided portion of the pill.
ALTERNATIVES

~ Avoid unnecessary induction
~ Avoid epidural anesthesia
~ Ask care provider if it is absolutely necessary.
~ Ask care provider if there are any alternatives.

Narcotics - Morphine, Stadol, Fentanyl, Nubain, etc.

Usually administered via the IV, narcotics go directly into the blood stream and to the baby. There is some measure of filtering by the placenta, however babies are effected by the medication.

"Virtually all drugs given during labor tend to cross the placenta rapidly and alter the fetal environment as they enter the circulatory system of the unborn infant within minutes or seconds of being administered to the mother" (Inch 1984:84).

Furthermore, the child's liver, which is one of the last organs to develop, must then detoxify their body from the drug. Keep in mind, the dosage given to a mother of 150 lbs is not appropriate for a child weighing only 7 lbs.

THE BENEFITS

~ Takes the "edge" off the pain
~ Allows mother to rest or sleep between contractions
~ May relieve anxiety and failure to progress

THE PROBLEMS

~ Mother still feels the full force of the contraction at it's peak, but does not feel the onset and departure of each
~ Requires someone to tell her the contraction is coming
~ May experience nausea
~ Mother feels less in control
~Sometimes a decrease in strength and frequency of contractions occurs temporarily

~ Depending on when given, may cause respiratory depression in the baby. If this occurs, an antidote can be administered and the side effects immediately reversed.
~ May cause the baby temporary difficulty with breastfeeding.
~ Requires IV administration
~ Requires bed rest
~ May have psychiatric side effects (see narcotic package insert)

"It will take the edge off of the pain"

Many are promised that narcotics will do just that, take the edge off. What they are not told, is which edge is taken off. Here is a contraction. Which part would you expect to be "taken off?"

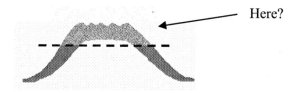

Here?

Actually, the top edge is not taken off, but rather the bottom edge is diminished, so that you will not be able to tell when a contraction is coming.

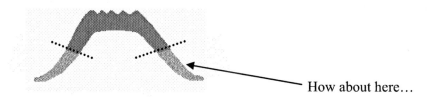

How about here…

You will need someone to watch the monitor to inform you so that you can brace yourself for a sudden peak of a contraction. With a natural contraction, you have the opportunity to work up to the peak, which allows you to control your ability to cope if it is an intense one. If you have had a narcotic, however, your contraction hits you full force and preparing to relax your body completely becomes very difficult while groggy, foggy, and nauseous.

Epidural Anesthesia

The epidural is regional anesthesia given via catheter inserted into the epidural space in the spinal column. If given properly, sensation below the injection site will be blocked, thus providing total pain relief.

THE BENEFITS

~ Does not alter the mother's consciousness
~ May provide a total block of all sensations below site
~ Can relax a mother with extreme anxiety
~ Can help lower blood pressure of a PIH patient
   (if blood platelets are high enough)

THE PROBLEMS

~ Completely immobilizes patient[6]
~ May have side effects
~ Patient no longer has an active role in the delivery of the baby[6]
~ Makes second stage longer and more difficult to push[7]
~ Increases the risk of vacuum or forceps assistance
~ Requires continuous electronic fetal monitoring
~ Requires an IV
~ Requires a urinary catheter
~ Requires a blood pressure cuff
~ Tubes, wires, and lines to strap you down in the bed
~ Risks of decreased blood pressure
~ May affect the baby's oxygen supply and affect his/her heart rate
~ Risks of causing more interventions especially if done too early
~ Risks of slowing down labor requiring pitocin[3]
~ Hypotension (drop in blood pressure)[1]
~ Inability to get a mal-positioned baby into place
~ Increased likelihood of the risk of vacuum extraction
~ Human error or abnormal spinal structure of the mother, such as inability to place catheter properly; inadvertent injection of anesthetic into a blood vessel; or too much anesthesia, affecting breathing and swallowing (Each anesthesiologist's skill level varies)

~ Increased likelihood of the need for an episiotomy
~ Fetal distress
~ Postpartum backache[4]
~ Urinary retention and postpartum urinary dysfunction[5]
~ Itching in the face, neck, and throat
~ Nausea and vomiting
~Spinal Headache – when there is a puncture in the spinal cord, and spinal fluid leaks back out, a thunderclap headache develops and you will not be able to sit up until it heals. Oftentimes, this requires yet another puncture to insert your own blood to "patch" the hole.
~Uncontrollable shivering
Uneven, incomplete or failed pain relief[1]
~ Postpartum feelings of regret
~Immobility that requires others to birth your baby for you
~Inability to push your baby out due to loss of perineal sensation, often requiring a cesarean section

Rare but Very Real and Serious Risks – They DO happen

~ Convulsions
~ Spinal cord damage, leading to paralysis
~ Cardiac arrest
~ Allergic shock
~ Epidural abscess
~ Respiratory arrest due to the epidural "going too high"
~ Maternal and/or fetal death
~ Possibility of low-grade fever - If membranes have been ruptured, the fever will have to be assumed to be caused by infection rather than epidural. Most care providers err on the side of caution - causing the baby to have to have a "septic work-up" for infection even though he/she is not infected
~ Can accidentally become a spinal if medication enters the dura space
~ May lead to the use of a urinary catheter, due to the fact the mom cannot get up to go to the bathroom.
~ Subtle short-term neurobehavioral effects up to six weeks of age, such as irritability and inconsolability and decreased ability to track an object visually or to shut out bright light and noise. There are no data on potential long-term effects.[1]
~ Possible difficulty with initial rooting and suckling behavior. Nurses have reported more difficulties in feeding medicated babies than unmedicated babies.

~ Interrupted mother-baby bonding time, due to reduced infant responsiveness. This may lead to long-term relationship difficulties.

ALTERNATIVES

~ Prayer
~ Hydrotherapy (water tubs, showers, warm foot soaks)
~ Bring a doula
~ Upright positions/out of bed
~ Massage
~ Birth room atmosphere
~ Supportive staff
~ Deep relaxation / Music therapy
~ Determination / Confident mindset
~ Counteract fear-tension-pain
~ Avoid unnecessary inductions and interventions
~ Maintain activity
~ Prenatal preparation (nutrition, exercise, education, practice)
~ Support from friends, family, and birth team
~ Faith in the body's ability to deliver a baby naturally

Episiotomy

A small incision in the perineum to facilitate the birth of the baby

- o Midline (Straight down)
- o Mediolateral (Diagonal)
- o "Hockey Stick" (Down and over)

THE BENEFITS

Opens an unusually tight perineum
Facilitates the birth when the baby is in distress
Shortens second stage labor
Easier for care provider to repair

THE PROBLEMS

Increased blood loss
Increased risk of a more serious tear (Most third degree tears happen after episiotomy)

Poor healing after delivery
   o   Natural tears zip back up and are less likely to break open
Longer healing period than a tear
More painful than a tear
Discomfort during intercourse
Pain at the site of the scar
Am J Obstet Gynecol. 1997 Feb;176(2):411-4

Most doctors do not, and should not, routinely practice episiotomy anymore, because it can cause serious damage to the perineum. Renew your mind in thinking that you will tear greatly if you don't get an episiotomy. Let's talk about tears.

First degree –	When only skin is separated
Second degree –	When skin and muscle are torn
Third degree –	When the perineal muscle is torn into the sphincter muscle
Fourth Degree –	When the tear extends all the way through the rectum

The majority of all third and fourth degree tears happen *after* an episiotomy is performed. It is like trying to tear a bed sheet. If you pull on it with your bare hands, it can be difficult. If, however, you snip a small cut, it rips very easily. Much the same, your tissue will be more likely to remain intact if you do not snip it.

The majority of serious tears that happen without an episiotomy are the result of poor management of the perineum. If a woman is lying on her back or semi-reclining, the baby's head is being pushed up and out, away from gravity against the perineum. This extra pressure is generally what causes a tear, because this is an unnatural position to be in. It is most convenient, of course, for the attendant to see what is going on. It is not the safest, however, because it pushes the tailbone and sacrum in the way of the space for the baby to come through, puts undue pressure causing a tear, etc.

If a woman is on her back while pushing, the attendant must be managing the perineum in order to prevent a tear. This takes skill, and physicians are now learning how to do that instead of cutting the tissue. It is much easier and safe, however, to be upright in a squat, or lying on one's side, so that the pressure on the skin is more natural.

Forceps

A tong-like instrument designed to clamp around fetal head in assistance of expedited delivery.

THE BENEFITS

Aids in speedy delivery in the event of a second stage delivery failure

THE PROBLEMS

~ Can cause maternal genital damage
~ Uterine rupture may occur
~ Can cause intracranial damage
~ Can cause fetal facial nerve damage
~ Lacerations of the face or scalp
~Can cause fractures of the face or skull

(World Heath Organization's guidelines)

Forceps Failed if:
1. Fetal head does not advance with each pull
2. Fetus is undelivered after three pulls with no descent or after 30 minutes
3. If there is no descent with every pull, discontinue
4. If forceps fail, a cesarean is required
5. Breaking the pubic symphysis is not an option if forceps fail

Vacuum Extraction

A soft bell-shaped and hemispheric silicone rubber cup is placed on the fetal head in an effort to facilitate delivery

THE BENEFITS

~ When mother is incapable of pushing the baby out (after an epidural, for example), the vacuum can assist in mechanically delivering the baby.
~ When the baby plummets into extreme distress (ie. below 60 bpm)and delivery needs to be hastened (tight knot in the cord, for example)

THE PROBLEMS

~ May cause fetal scalp laceration if twisted
~ May cause a cephalohematoma (1-26% of vacuum assisted deliveries)
~ May cause eye hemorrhaging
~ Intracranial hemorrhage (has been found to occur in one of every 860 vacuum deliveries)
~ May cause damage to maternal tissue
~ May cause fetal death

ALTERNATIVES

~ Avoid an epidural
~ Avoid exhaustion
~ Get in a squat to open pelvic outlet more
~ Try different positions

Cesarean Section

The extraction of the fetus by means of surgical incision to the abdomen

Incision types
   o   Vertical incision
       Used in an emergent situation
       More likely to rupture in subsequent deliveries
   o   Bikini incision
       Horizontal incision low in the abdomen
               Incision is less likely to rupture in subsequent deliveries

Reasons for Cesarean

   o   Cervical dystocia (failure to progress)
       Often caused by tension/anxiety
       Fetal Distress
   o   Mal-presentation (position of the baby is not ideal)

o Abruptio placenta (placenta detaches from uterus prematurely) Immediate need for c-section
o Placenta previa (placenta has grown over the opening of the uterus/cervix)
o Partial or complete at term pregnancy
o Early pregnancy - can rectify itself
o Active herpes lesion
o Cord prolapse (umbilical cord drops out of the uterus before the baby is born)
o Cephalo-pelvic disproportion (CPD) (Baby's head is too big to come out of the pelvis) Squatting can open pelvic outlet by 1cm
o Pregnancy Induced Hypertension (toxemia)
o Multiple babies
o Deformity with the baby

THE BENEFITS

~ Can be life saving
~ Date of delivery can be scheduled

THE PROBLEMS

~ Baby does not benefit from the pressure of the vaginal
canal squeezing amniotic fluid out of the lungs
~ Baby does not benefit from being exposed to beneficial bacteria that would otherwise colonize in the gut, preventing many food allergies and diarrhea later in life.
~ Interference with normal breastfeeding
~ Possible infection
~ Increased risk of blood clots in the legs, pelvic organs
and sometimes lungs
~ Maternal death
~ Major abdominal surgery
~ Interference with normal bonding time

All of these procedures have their place when indicated, meaning that there is medical reason to use them. It is important to completely understand the risks prior to giving consent to the procedure. Sometimes decisions for intervention are made as a precautionary measure, due to a possibility that something *may* go wrong in the future.

If you are presented with one of these aforementioned interventions, you might want to ask your care provider the following questions:

1. Is my baby okay?
2. Am I okay?
3. What would happen if we waited an hour and tried something non-clinical first?
4. Do you have any suggestions for alternatives?
5. What are ALL the risks of this procedure?

If the mother and baby are okay, then it might be feasible to try alternatives for a while to see if a solution can be found naturally in order to avoid intervention, using it only as a last resort. In order to be able to have the knowledge and skills needed to achieve natural childbirth, the parents should make every effort to prepare themselves. They can do this by going to a good childbirth education class that has a high natural childbirth rate. A good class is small in size, and long in length, spending adequate time on coaching techniques and comfort measures.

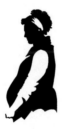

1. Avard, D.M., and Nimroof, C.M. "Risks and Benefits of Obstetrical Epidural Analgesia: A Review." *Birth* 12(4):215-225, Winter, 1985.
2. Lester, B.M., Als, H., Brazelton, T.B. "Regional Obstetric Anesthesia and Newborn Behavior: A Reanalysis Toward Synergistic Effects." *Child Development* 53:687-692, 1982
3. Thorp, J.A., Parisi, V.M., Boylan, P.C., Johnston, D.A. "The Effect of Continuous Epidural Analgesia on Cesarean Section for Dystocia in Nulliparous Women." *American Journal of Obstetrics and Gynecology* 161(3):670-675, September 1989.4. MacArthur, C., Lewis, M., Knox, E.G., and Crawford, J.S. "Epidural Anesthesia and Long-Term Backache After Childbirth." *British Medical Journal*, 301:9-12, July 7, 1990. 5. Dickersin, K. "Pharmacological Control of Pain During Labor." In: Chalmers, I., Enkin, M., Keirse, M., eds, *Effective Care in Pregnancy and Childbirth*. New York: Oxford University Press, 1989. 6. McKay, S., and Roberts, J. "Obstetrics by Ear," *American Journal of Midwifery* 35(5):266-273, Sept/Oct 1990. 7. Maresh, M., Choong, K.H., and Beard, R.W. "Delayed Pushing with Lumbar Epidural Analgesia in Labour." *British Journal Obstetrics and Gynaecology* 90(7):623-627, July 1983.

Bible Study Discussion

1. How serious are you in achieving natural childbirth?

2. What have you done to further study interventions and their pros/cons?

3. What have you done to prepare for natural childbirth?

4. Have you talked with your care-provider to make sure you are on the same page regarding your birth plan?

5. What part of this chapter stands out to you?

Chapter Fifteen
Bible Stories and Birth

Now Jabez was more honorable than his brothers,
and his mother called his name Jabez, saying, "Because
I bore him in pain." And Jabez called on the God of Israel
saying, "Oh, that You would bless me indeed, and enlarge
my territory, that Your hand would be with me, and that
You would keep me from evil, that I may not cause pain!"
So God granted him what he requested.
1 Chronicles 4:9 – 10 (NKJV)

This recently popular prayer is hidden in a sea of genealogy, deep in the depths of otherwise painfully boring accounts of family members who bore so-in-so, and they bore this guy, who was the father of that man, who begat this person, and so on. I remember trying to read the New Testament from the beginning as a young girl, only to be snagged by the genealogy in the first chapter of Matthew. Time after time, I would just toss it back on the shelf, never accomplishing my goal.

To my delight, however, a wise Pastor explained to us one night that the family lines in that chapter, when studied, reveal that the blood-line from David to Jesus contains some not-so-honorable folks. One might expect a king to be of a quality pedigree with nothing but proud history - seemingly out of reach for common folk. Part of the lovely nature of Jesus Christ, however, is that He is a humble King, willing to associate Himself with the even the lowliest, who can relate to Him as an approachable and dear friend.

Although the beginning of the book of Matthew might indeed be yawn-invoking, hidden within the genealogy is a rich and beautiful truth that makes it come alive to anyone willing to examine it deeper. The Bible is filled with these hidden jewels that are there for the spiritual archaeologist to uncover.

If scripture is viewed as a living document, one that can be applied to any application in life, then even those seeking wisdom about childbirth can be encouraged and directed by the stories and accounts. The Christian looks to the New Testament for stories about the Savior, but a careful dig through the ancient Old Testament would reveal Jesus on nearly every page as well.

For example, when studying Numbers chapter two, one might argue that it is quite possibly the most boring chapter in the Bible. Here you have the census of all of the tribes. It details where they put their camps, geographically, in respect to each other. This is how the Lord instructed them to live, according to His word given to Moses and Aaron.

Amazingly, this story is an example of how the Lord has encrypted His plan for salvation within the records of His people. God asked the children of Israel to camp in a certain geographical setup; certain tribes to the North of the Levites, other tribes to the South, East, and West. Each tribe varied in their size, so there was not an equal amount of people on each side of the Levites. If a person were to fly in an airplane and pass over the camps of the children of Israel, they would see a most amazing sight. These camps would be configured in the shape of – a cross!

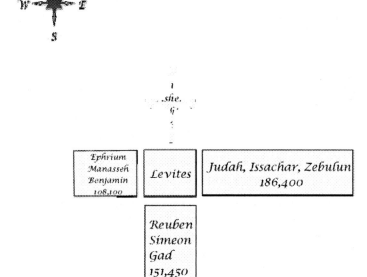

The cross was not upright as you think it would be, however. It was on its side with the top of it pointing west. Why in the world would the Lord have the cross on its side? Consider this. The children of Israel were traveling west, in the direction of their promised land. God may have been saying - because the people were traveling toward the promised land in the shape of a cross, the way to the ultimate promised land (Heaven) would be achieved by the cross of Calvary! What a fantastic story! Much the same, this Biblical birth story gives us a glimpse into the anthropology of birth in Old Testament Biblical times. Have we evolved so much since then that these principles cannot be applied to us?

Jabez and Birth

This text tells us that Jabez had at least two other siblings. Because the author used the word brothers as plural, we know that his mother had at least three children. What is noteworthy is that she specifically gave Jabez his name because for that birth, she experienced unusual pain. Jabez, literally translated, means "he causes pain" (NKJV). It is therefore safe to assume that the other two brothers were birthed more easily and with less pain.

We do not know exactly how much pain she experienced with the rest of her children, but it is clear that the birth of Jabez was one of sorrow. I point this out because many in Western society are convinced that each and every birth is destined to be excruciating, painful, and something to be feared. However, here we have an example that illustrates for us that a painful birth (like that of Jabez's) is actually out of the ordinary and not the normal course of events for the people of the Bible.

What can we learn from the mother of Jabez? Painful and difficult births were not the norm, and uneventful births seemed to be the everyday occurrence during the Biblical times. Having a baby can at times be troublesome and very painful, but we are not cursed to endure undue hardship with each and every child that is born.

Western thought tends to reverse that thinking, who has been treating childbirth as an illness. Because we think that way, are we not creating a self-fulfilling prophecy? It is true that most Western women are not able to cope with the toils of delivery, and need some sort of medical assistance to get through. Could it be that much of the technology that is used is a result of the complications that arise from simple fear?

It is this fear that can lead a woman down the road to excruciating pain, thus making labor a medical event. By eliminating fear and replacing it with confidence and understanding, much of the intervention used would be deemed unnecessary and the normal course of labor would be tolerable by the majority of women.

Enlarging Your Territory

In a figurative sense, we can ask God to enlarge the "territory" of our pain threshold. Any intervention carries with it potential risks, and because we love our babies, we would not want to be irresponsible and use them unless there was absolute need. In order to get through childbirth, we need to ask God to enlarge the territory of our capacity to manage the pain in other ways.

Going back and looking at the prayer again, you'll notice that Jabez fervently cried out to the Lord. "Oh, Lord, that you would bless me indeed!" was his request. We need to get to a place where we desperately desire that the Lord would bless us with the peace that we need to achieve confidence during childbirth. This prayer needs to be prayed long before we go into labor so that we can continue to seek His guidance before labor begins.

In a literal sense, it is almost humorous to think about. Yet during childbirth, we can pray this prayer and mean it! "Lord, enlarge my territory," you might exclaim! The territory, of course, would be the cervix and/or the vaginal outlet. Asking the Lord to enlarge that territory so that you might not cause or feel unnecessary pain is perfectly okay!

The Bible certainly is a living document almost breathing with life. Once a person decides to delve deeply into the riches of God's word, it becomes like one of those novels that you just cannot put down. Except, it isn't a novel at all, but factual history that we can apply to our daily lives, even childbirth. Jesus Christ can be found on each and ever page if we look for Him, and He desires to bless us so that we might live life to the fullest.

Bible Study Discussion

1. Where has God made Himself known to you in your life?

2. What do you think about Jabez's birth being more painful than his brothers? Why was it notable enough to name him that?

3. Where else in the Old Testament does it point to Christ? (For example, Isaiah 53)

4. How did Rachel's birth of Benjamin compare to Jabez's birth?

5. What part of this chapter stands out to you?

Chapter Sixteen
The "Natural Childbirth" Tool Box

Nevertheless she will be saved in childbearing
if they continue in faith, love, and holiness, with self-control.
1 Timothy 2:15 (NKJV)

Each woman carries in her own mind the ideal components that would make the birth of her child a fabulous event. For some, a great birth equates to having a room full of family and friends to witness the birth of their baby. For others, it may be that they only want their husband present, because to them, birth is a very private thing. Some desire to birth in the comfort of their own home, while others prefer to deliver in the hospital. The perception of what an ideal birth experience is can be as varied as the fingerprints on our fingers. This chapter will be devoted to those who desire to achieve a birth that is free of medical intervention; or in other words, natural childbirth.

For the Christian, the process is entirely different. The *world* tells us that we should "birth from within," finding our strength inside ourselves. They teach that the women who achieve natural childbirth are "strong women" with a high tolerance for pain.

For the believer, however, our glory is in our weakness, and our strength is in our Creator. Now we no longer have to rely on our threshold of pain and ability to cope, but on the One whose yoke is easy and whose burden is light. Jesus sent us a Comforter so that we can surrender control to God, being comforted as we bring forth our child. In surrendering, birth often becomes bearable. The scriptures tell us exactly how to do just that.

The scripture listed at the beginning of the chapter contains all the elements needed to achieve birth naturally. We will take each component and expound on it, in an effort to give you some tools to take with you. Notice that it says "if *they* continue" not "if *she* continues." Both husband and wife need to walk in this way for her to receive the blessing promised in this verse. I encourage husbands to study this section, pray it in, and then be available for their wives during the birth of their child. She needs you!

Benefits of Natural Childbirth

- Safety – Natural childbirth has consistently been shown to be the safest method of delivery there is. Infant and maternal mortality rates are lower in natural births. Few are trained in undisturbed natural childbirth management, so if you want true support, ensure your attendants know how to help you.
- Prevention Model of Care – Providers who are interested in helping you achieve natural childbirth will be working with you from the beginning of pregnancy to help you realize a natural birth through diet, exercise, and education.
- Early Family Bonding – Families who have a natural birth are more likely to have a healthy bonding period in the immediate postpartum. Babies are more likely to be alert and responsive immediately after birth. Mothers who deliver naturally are more likely to have a better breastfeeding experience.
- Confidence – Parents who deliver naturally tend to gain increased confidence in themselves.
- Patience – Mothers who learn relaxation and coping techniques during labor utilize those techniques in a myriad of situations required of parents later in the child's life.
- Shorter Labors – Many interventions can slow down and even stop labor. This usually begins the cascade of intervention in order to medically manage the birth that now has become abnormal.
- Faster recovery – A mom who births naturally is less likely to hemorrhage, tear, have postpartum infections, and other complications after birth. She will tend to feel little or no pain after the baby is born, in contrast to medicated and surgical births.
- Easier Transition to Breast Feeding – Babies who are not drugged, groggy, or separated early in the immediate postpartum will tend to have a greater instinct to find the breast and latch sooner.
- Less expensive – Obviously, a natural birth will cost dramatically less than a medical birth. Once one medical domino is fallen, many other very expensive procedures will more than likely follow.

- Satisfaction – Most mothers who achieve natural childbirth say that it was the most wonderful experience in their life and they look forward to doing it again.
- Sacrificial love – Because interventions carry with them real risks, we have the opportunity to deny ourselves and strive for a pure labor for the sake of our child.

Continuing in Faith

Before we can tackle natural childbirth, we have to have the faith that it can be done. In the Western world, that task seems next to impossible! We have just about everyone telling us that it *cannot* be done. The television says so, and many often suggest that it is no longer necessary. Our friends tell us how wonderful the pain medication is and how horrible their labor was without it.

Redefining Normal Birth

How do we undo the years of influence that defines what birth is in our minds? Romans 12:2 says, "Do not conform any longer to the pattern of this world, but be transformed by the renewing of your mind." Our thoughts can be transformed by changing our outlook on how we were created – created to give birth! We no longer focus on the pain-increasing fear of giving birth, but on the faith that we have in God's design.

If we lack faith, we can remember that God said that He is faithful, even when we are faithless. We know that we have been created to deliver children, and we also know that sometimes things come up that cause us to rely on the care of others. We can trust God that He has given us the tools to handle the tough situations, thus allowing ourselves to let go and give birth!

Continuing in Love

Greater love has no man than this,
that a man lay down his life for his friends.
John 15:13

Jesus sets the example for us at the Mount of Olives on the night He was to be arrested. The Messiah clearly chose to endure the pain of the cross, even though He himself was apprehensive and fearful to the point of hematidrosis, a condition which causes rupture of the surface capillaries when under extreme stress. Luke tells us in his gospel that Jesus' sweat was like drops of blood falling to the ground, indicating that He was under an enormous amount of anguish. He prayed earnestly that night for God to save Him from the cross, but was willing to do what God asked of Him, despite His own desires.

Once on the cross, He was offered a sip of wine vinegar (some say it was used in those days as pain relief) to help ease the anquish, but refused it. Although we are not told why He did, we might guess that Jesus did not want to diminish the suffering that He was under as He completed the work of salvation for all who believe.

The book of Hebrews tells us that Jesus endured the cross out of the joy that was set before Him. This is much like a laboring woman who endures the pain of labor, knowing that there is pure joy coming once her baby arrives. Many women who have delivered their babies both naturally and with medication will tell you that the great joy of delivery was magnified after having struggled through the hard work of labor.

The most common reason that parents attempt natural childbirth, however, is for the benefit of the baby. It is undeniable that any intervention carries with it some measure of risk. I cannot imagine any person that would partake of an intervention for the sole purpose of putting their child in danger; it just does not happen. The reason we do elect to take medication, of course, is to alleviate fear and to make it more comfortable "for us."

"For our _light_ affliction, which is but for a moment, is working for us a far more exceeding and eternal weight of glory..."
II Corinthians 4:17

It is true that this "light affliction" is only temporary and for only a moment in time. The parents who attempt natural childbirth try to walk in love for their child, putting needs and desires aside for the benefit of an unborn life. Let love be the second tool utilized in resisting the urge to eliminate the discomfort of bringing forth our new family member.

Continuing in Holiness

Let us fix our eyes upon Jesus, the author and perfecter of our faith,
who for the joy set before him endured the cross, despising its shame,
and sat down at the right hand of the throne of God.
Hebrews 12:2

The word holy is defined as being complete, lacking nothing. We fall short of the glory of holiness, and therefore we look to Jesus to be One who completes our faith. Once we have Him, we can go into the delivery room with the confidence that He will provide for our every need. Those who attend the Christ-centered childbirth will notice that something is very different than the average run-of-the-mill birth. The Holy Spirit guides us in ways that cause us to be effective witnesses to those who observe us. If we are acting in a way that is less than holy, then we cannot represent Christ to the person attending us that never knew Him. Every word that is said, every action that is exhibited, needs to be taken captive and made obedient to Christ.

Another aspect to holiness during childbirth is the condition of our minds, and the effect that narcotics has on us. The Bible teaches us that when we surrender control to a mind-altering drug, the possibility for the influence of the unholy increases. In Biblical times, the sorcerers would administer these drugs to people making them more susceptible to the magic that they employed. Today, people use these drugs as recreation, and the demonic effect that it has on them is undisputable. Because of the evil that is associated with mind-altering drugs, parents may want to use extreme caution when electing to alleviate pain with narcotics.

Pharmakeia, where we get the word pharmaceutical, in and of itself is not unholy. It is the effect of Satan on a vulnerable mind that is what we try to avoid. He desires to instill guilt, insecurity, accusations, etc into the minds of those involved. Better to not give him a foothold by maintaining a sober mind than to receive a narcotic that really isn't that effective in the first place.

In all aspects of labor and delivery, we should try to continue in holiness. That might mean keeping ourselves from bitter language, uncontrolled, or unholy behavior. Above all, we aim to continue in a sober state of mind, our third tool that motivates us to achieve a medication-free childbirth.

*Notwithstanding, she shall be saved in childbearing, if they
continue in faith and charity and holiness with <u>sobriety</u>.
1 Timothy 2:15 (King James Version)*

Continuing With Self-Control

*So then, let us not be like others, who are asleep,
but let us be alert and self-controlled.
1 Thessalonians 5:6*

Like a long-distance runner, women in labor need to employ endurance, discipline, and self-control, if they desire to go through it without drugs. Physical strength is needed, but even more important than this is the need to be mentally ready. The interpretation of sensations, mental activity, and determination are the hallmarks of a disciplined mind.

Interpretation of Sensations

Enlarging your threshold of pain means redefining how you interpret what you are feeling. This is quite simple and anybody can achieve it if they purpose to try. All it takes is an incident that would normally cause you to cringe in pain. For instance, if you stub your toe on a kitchen chair, instead of biting your lip and hopping on the other foot, try taking in several cleansing breaths and deciding that it is not pain that you feel, but rather a different sensation altogether. Feel the tingling that is happening, the pulsing of your vein, and all the other sensations that come along with it, but leave out the "ouch." You will find that each time you are better able to cope with the pain and reframe it into a different interpretation.

Activity To Try:

Go to the ice box and take out a piece of ice, making sure it doesn't stick to your skin! Hold it in your hand for sixty seconds. (Don't read ahead until after you have done this)...

For most people, holding a piece of ice for sixty seconds gets very uncomfortable, very fast. Next, get another piece of ice, but this time as it melts in your <u>other</u> hand, take deep abdominal breaths like you learned how to do earlier in the book, and change the way you interpret the sensations, as you relax your shoulders and all of your muscles, breathing abdominally. You will find that it is much easier to get through the sixty seconds as you interpret the cold sensation in an entirely new light.

Even the keenest of minds, however, may begin to break down during an unusually difficult childbirth. The beautiful thing about this is that God designed us to need each other, and when this situation occurs, the role of the birth coach is most important. He or she can pray for you, help you to stay focused, and give you the support and encouragement needed to get you through the tough spots.

Mental Activity

God made us to want some sort of predictability during labor. Many women will form a "routine" as they cope with the contractions. Frequently it is swaying the hips back and forth (a great way to help the baby come down), making deep, open-throated vocal tones, looking at a particular focal point, or breathing in a prescribed manner. For the Christian, the number one routine that can be employed is that of a memorized prayer, especially if it is one that she has created herself. By greeting each contraction with prayerful meditation, a healthy pattern develops, creating a predictability that is very comforting.
Here is an example:

Father God, thank you for this contraction, for it will bring me one step closer to holding my baby. Body, in the name of Jesus Christ, remain as relaxed as possible. I give myself permission to open up and let my baby out, Lord. Guard my heart and my mind from the darts of the enemy, and keep me holy. Lord, enlarge the territory of my flesh and allow my baby to come out with the least amount of pain possible. Let the labor be quick, Lord, but not too quick that it would hurt my child. Let all things happen in your perfect timing and according to your will. In Jesus' name, Amen.

It is so tempting to allow our thoughts to go from peace to tension as the pressure of the uterus contracting intensifies. We might hear ourselves thinking, "I can't do this, this hurts, make it stop." When this begins to happen, we can follow the example of Paul and the church of Corinth who claimed, "We take every thought captive, to make it obedient to Christ. (2 Corinthians 10:5)." The negative thoughts are taken "captive" and placed in the dungeon of our mind, so that they can no longer torture us. These are the very thoughts that will cause the sympathetic nervous system to respond by stalling the labor with painful resistance from the inner muscle layer of the uterus.

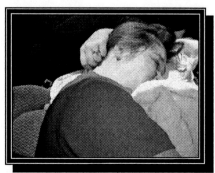

Courtesy of Jennifer Vanderlaan

Determination

If we don't determine to birth naturally, and we are given a long and difficult labor, then it becomes almost an insurmountable task. Where does the determination come from? For some, it is because a friend was able to do it, and they want to be able to do it too. For many, it is the fear of needles. For most, it is out of care and concern for the baby. Whatever the reason, we need to ultimately be aware of the risks of any medical procedure.

A thirsty search for the truth of each intervention and the risks and benefits they offer should begin long before the due date approaches. Decisions made out of emotion are nothing more than irresponsible and dangerous. As God's children, we have an obligation to the child (of whom He has given us custody) to seek the truth in all the procedures that could potentially be performed. Often the truth about these procedures should be motivation enough to give us the determination to do without.

Fundamentally, you will need the support from those around you. If your attendants are offering you something to "take the edge off" at a time that you are vulnerable, you may not be able to endure the difficult moments of labor. Let them know in early labor that you do not want them to offer medication. If things get too intense, try something different from what you are doing. Are you totally alert? Then try to go into a very deep state of relaxation so that you can cope better.

Means to an End

- Determination – You must have a solid purpose for wanting to achieve natural childbirth and stick to it.
- Your support team (professional doula)
- Good childbirth education (Bradley classes, or a class specific to natural birth)
- Self-education
- Your care provider must be supportive, and experienced in hands-off management of labor
- Your personal fitness and diet must be polished
- Support from friends/family
- Spirituality must be strong, placing all trust in your Creator to achieve what you were formed to do – to give birth!
- Your mental health must be nurtured. If there is any former abuse, you must come to terms with that, separating the birth experience and know that it is a completely different situation. This time, make it your day that you control, with a wonderful gift after it is completed – a baby of your own to love, teach, and protect!
- Practice – this is imperative. Abdominal breathing, mind control, muscle control, positioning during contractions, prayer, etc are all things to have practiced amply before labor begins
- Fathers prepared – Dads can be an enormous help during birth, and need to be practicing as well.
- Attitude – Fear will make the process more painful, even unbearable. You must be confident and feel safe where you birth for things to go normally.
- Knowledge of the risks of interventions. This is perhaps the most important aspect of natural childbirth. Be thorough in your quest for truth in this matter.

It is important to remember that there is no one right way to give birth. We were not created as machines that have babies exactly alike and any divergence means that we failed. God made each woman unique, and each woman's own births unique. There is a lesson to be learned from each birth that is applicable to our own life. We only have to have the eyes to look for that lesson that God is trying to show us.

The Lord, I believe, does allow for a little control on our part over how our labor is managed. Although He has a plan for our birth,

He is gracious and merciful and gives us a measure of control that can affect the events of the delivery. Satan, too, is right there planning on how to infiltrate our experience and destroy it. Take the information presented in this book, steeped in much prayer, and trust in the Lord's Romans 8:28 promise that says that all things happen for a good reason. With that in mind, you will be better equipped to surrender your fear to Him and allow His beautiful work to be done!

Bible Study Discussion

1. Has your perception of natural childbirth changed?

2. What do you think natural childbirth will be like?

3. Is it possible for a person to have an enjoyable birth naturally?

4. If you have decided to have a medicated birth, have you researched every possible fact regarding the risks of each intervention?

5. Have you completed your birth plan?

Chapter Seventeen
Coaching Techniques

Coaches, she needs you during labor. Each woman will define how much she needs you, but know that at whatever level, she will benefit from your presence. You are her anchor, her guide, her protector, her strong tower, her refuge and her sanctuary. Prepare to involve yourself to the fullest extent that she will need you. Expect to engage in your own labor of love, forsaking all others while you and she bring forth a new life.

The coach's task can be daunting and uncertain, and you may be feeling a little insecure at your ability to help when things really get going. Just as she needs to set her fears aside to avoid unnecessary pain, you will also need to resist the temptation of fleeing the scene. Many coaches have gone before you, and many have felt helpless and alone. Thanks be to God that you are a believer in the Holy Spirit who leads you in confidence.

Fathers, you have a fantastic opportunity to build your marriage during childbirth, as the labor process can do one of two things: it can bind you with a holy glue that nothing can separate, or it can drive a cold wedge between you and your wife. It may be tempting to retreat from the situation and go within yourself or perhaps maybe even leave the room. Fight that urge and overcome it like your wife overcomes her contractions and press on towards your goal of being a supportive husband. You won't regret it!

This chapter will equip you with some ideas and tools to help her during all phases of labor. Bring this book with you to the birth in case you forget something when things get heavy.

Father, You are awesome beyond all of our imagination. Thank you for giving this couple the opportunity to share in Your creation of life. Strengthen them, bind their hearts, and give them Your Holy Spirit to guide them. Go before them, come up behind them, and place a hedge of protection on all sides of them. Strengthen this coach with godly leadership and courage, and take away any doubt or fear that might creep up on him during the process. May he not feel helpless, because he has You on his side. Give him wisdom and power for this time. In Jesus' name, Amen!

Early Labor

Recognizing Early Labor

- Emotionally excited, joyful, talkative, needing to be busy.
- She should be able to talk through the contractions.
- Contractions are usually irregular and at least 5 minutes apart.
- The cervix is between 0 and 3 centimeters
- Contractions usually last 30 seconds or less.
- The cervix is usually posterior or "hard to reach."

Note: Not all labors follow the typical course, and we can never assume that she is in early labor without knowing the dilation and position of the cervix. However, the sooner she is in the hospital, the more likely she is to have interventions.

Things To Do

- Make sure the bag is packed
- Get all the baby items into the car (especially the infant car seat).
- Make sure that she is not alone (If you must leave for a short time, get someone to stay with her).
- Suggest that she engage in an activity if it is during the day, or try to sleep if it is at night
- Time contractions (start of one to the start of the next) but do not become preoccupied with them
- Contact your provider to inform them about the events that are happening
- Contact your doula
- Maintain normal activity
- Get something to eat for you both & keep her hydrated

Things To Bring To The Hospital

- Bible
- Prenatal reports and insurance information
- Comfortable night robe & slippers

- Hairbrush, curling iron, hairdryer, shampoo, makeup, and toiletries
- Camera & video equipment
- Phone card
- Hand-held fan
- Clothes to go home in (what she wore at six months pregnant) / Car seat
- Baby clothes (no gowns with drawstring as it is hard to buckle in the car seat)
- Snacks, but take care to notice your oral hygiene (she is VERY sensitive to odor)
- Cotton underwear (several pairs), sanitary pads & Nursing Bra (at least two)
- Eye glasses (if needed)
- Small amount of money
- Aroma therapy (candles may not be permitted due to oxygen tank & flame hazard)
- Massage tools & massage oil or lotion/tennis ball
- Rice sock (Fill a tube sock with rice and tie a knot. Microwave for two minutes and use as a hot compress – lavender may be added for aroma)
- Raw honey (processed honey is nothing more than sugar)
- Favorite music & music player

Active Labor

Recognizing Active Labor

- She can talk between contractions, but may need to pause during one.
- She is getting more serious and less willing to socialize.
- Contractions are usually regular and at no more than 5 minutes apart.
- The cervix is usually between 4 – 6 centimeters.
- Contractions usually last 45 - 60 seconds.
- The cervix begins to move forward.
- The head of the baby may be getting deeper in the pelvis.

Things To Do

- Most important, make sure that she remains relaxed and confident.
- Help establish her nest by dimming the lights, establishing privacy, putting on soft worship music, limiting visitors and noise, and help her stay comfortable.
- Give her a massage. Long, complete strokes from the top of the shoulder and all the way down past the fingers is better than rubbing the middle of her upper arm. All strokes should be downward. On her back, start at the top with both hands and rub all the way down her spine and then when you get to her hips widen the stroke like an upside down funnel. Don't forget to give her a foot massage!
- Make sure she changes positions every hour.
- Make sure she urinates every two hours.
- Keep her well hydrated, taking a sip of water or juice after each contraction.
- Make sure she takes in some sort of calories, such as fruit juice or raw honey.
- Keep her in an upright position, moving if possible.
- Keep small talk to a minimum, as it distracts her from focusing on relaxing.
- Help her begin to enter into a state of deep relaxation and tranquility.
- Lead her in prayer or communion.
- Suggest getting into the tub. If she cannot, try the shower. If the shower is out of the question, then perhaps a warm foot-soak while in the rocking chair. Use hydrotherapy wherever possible.
- Watch for tension in her hands, brow, jaw, arms, back, etc.
  If you see tension, touch her there gently and say soothing words like, "Let go right here."
  (Try not to use the word "relax")

- Maintain constant physical contact with her (holding her hand during a contraction, moving her hair out of her face, gentle massage, eye contact, etc.) unless she does not want to be touched. Never leave her alone. If you need to eat, have someone bring it to you and eat in the room. If you need to use the restroom, use the one in the room. If you need to rest, use the chair or bench provided in the room. If you must leave the room, do it for the absolute least amount of time and have a doula or friend replace you.
- Ask her if she has discomfort in her lower back. If so, offer counter pressure right above the "crack" in her buttocks. A firm, steady pressure is better than massage.

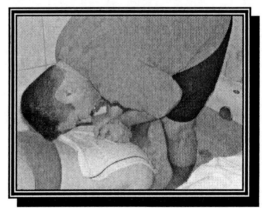

"A Good Laugh During Hard Work"
Taken by Maureen Johnston & Monique Micallef

- Encourage her routine (belly dancing, rocking, counting, etc.)
- Encourage her to enter into a deep rest.
- Make sure that your needs are being met.

If pain becomes unbearable:

- Suggest the jacuzzi or shower.
- Try a position change.
- Increase your level of support for her (May need to use a gentle authoritative approach)
- Remind her of the "second wind" of endorphins.

- Make sure she is in a tranquil state – a state of heightened alertness makes it difficult to cope with the waves of contractions.
- Help her focus on just one contraction at a time.
- Don't discuss anything during the contraction, wait until it is over. Say, "Lets just get through this contraction and then we can talk about it afterwards."
- Is she in bed? Get her up to her feet and do the slow dance position with someone giving her counter pressure on her back as they give her an arm massage.
- Remind her of how strong she is, and tell her she has more strength inside of her.
- Give gentle but constant eye contact, and do shallow abdominal breathing with her. Simply say, "Breathe with me, breathe with me. Like this, yes….that's it….good, good for you. Stay on top of it, stay on top of it… it's coming down now, almost gone, now just rest. Good job, honey! I love you!)

Transition

Recognizing Transition

- May become insecure, unsure, may desire to escape the pain.
- She usually will not want to talk at all, unless absolutely necessary.
- Anything that distracts her from her total focus on relaxation is unwelcome.
- Contractions are one right after another, usually about 1-2 minutes apart.
- The cervix is between 7 – 10 centimeters.
- Contractions usually last 60-90 seconds.
- She may tremble, vomit, get too hot and too cold, or feel like she has to have a bowel movement.
- The head of the baby may be getting deeper in the pelvis.

Things To Do:

- Remind her of how far she has come.
- Everything that you were doing for active labor, except you will be increasing your level of support.

- Help her convert to a more shallow abdominal breathing.
- Fan her during contractions, keep her warm between them according to her comfort level.
- Check her mental state ("What was going through your mind during that last contraction?").
- Watch for tension in her hands, brow, jaw, arms, back, etc. Tell her lovingly, "It is really important for you to stay confident and loose now. You don't want to get 'stuck' at 8 cm!"
- If you see tension, touch her there gently and say soothing words like, "Let go right here." **(Try not to use the word "relax" or "breathe")**
- Maintain constant physical contact with her.
- Do not leave her now.
- Make sure she has some caloric intake to prepare for pushing.
- Stay close to her face.

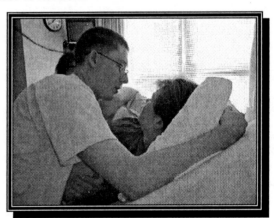

Courtesy of Jennifer Vanderlaan

- Keep her out of bed.
- Try the jacuzzi now if you haven't already.
- Remind her that if she takes narcotics now, the baby is likely to be born groggy.
- Remind her that she is almost there.
- Do not get involved in small talk that takes your attention away from mom. Learn to allow long periods of silence. Or on the other hand, if she needs you to talk during the contraction, develop a soothing set of things to say in rhythm with her breathing.

- Most importantly, don't panic. It is difficult to see your loved one in pain, and it is very tempting to want to "rescue" her from it. It is quite normal for a woman to get very agitated or upset, to cry out, and to act in great despair during transition. Although this doesn't always happen, as some women are so relaxed that the staff is surprised to find out that they are so far along in the labor.

- If she was determined before labor to do it naturally, she will need you now more than ever to be strong and help her through this. Check with the nurse that the baby's heart tones are fine and that the mother is fine. If so, then take heart that this is the most intense part of labor, and it is almost over. When second stage comes, it most likely will feel much different and perhaps better while she is pushing. If she wants drugs, remind her it is too close to the birth and narcotics will affect the baby and an epidural will affect her ability to push. She's almost there! Don't give up on her!

Second Stage (Pushing)

How to recognize when she is beginning second stage labor

- Sometimes women get a 15-30 minute break in contractions before it is time to push. Many women have unnecessarily received pitocin during this time, while at ten centimeters without contractions. Use this time to regroup and regain strength for second stage.

- She may announce to you that she has to go to the bathroom at some point past 7 centimeters. Ask her if it is to urinate or to have a bowel movement. If she says it is to have a bowel movement, then you will need to let the nurse or provider know because oftentimes this is the baby's head pressing on the nerves in the rectum that alert her to use the bathroom. This is a sign that the baby has descended into the vagina and second stage is getting closer or imminent.

- Be listening for a little "catch" in the breath while she is exhaling. The urge to grunt can be as small as a break in the exhalation, or detectable as a loud grunt in the midst of a very vocal contraction. The vocal moan changes to more of an uncontrollable primal grunt that is unmistakable of second stage

231

pushing. The nurse will most likely be coming in on her own after hearing this!

- She may open those once tranquil eyes with a look of panic and an emphatic, "Help me!" Some women are frightened by the change in sensations of second stage contractions. This is normal and your reassurance that everything is fine will help her tremendously.

Things To Do:

- Begin preparing for the tasks of second stage.
- Get ice chips, fan, cool cloth, chap stick, camera, etc. ready.
- Prepare a basin of extra warm water and a get a stack of wash cloths.
  for perineal hot compresses (Check with nurse first).
- Get her some sort of juice or tea with raw honey for glucose (not orange juice).
- Grab an orange juice for yourself, you'll need the extra energy now.
- Talk about what position she wants to birth in and help her get into it. Remember, it is difficult to verbalize what they want, and even more difficult to move. You will really have to help her and perhaps even speak for her during this time.
- Check her mental state (What was going through your mind during that last contraction?)
- Watch for apprehension of second stage. Many women are fearful of pushing.
- Remind her to drop her bottom down and open during a push.
- Make sure she is breathing adequately. Say, "Deep breath in for your baby" right before she is going to push.
- Praise her sincerely.
- Maintain constant physical contact with her (holding her leg during a
  contraction, for example) unless she does not want to be touched.
- Encourage her to remain in a deep rest between contractions.
- Pay attention to your hygiene. Laboring women are very sensitive to odor.
- Do not get involved in small talk that takes your attention away from mom.

- Learn to allow long periods of silence between contractions.
- Speak gently and quietly, she will hear you best this way. Stay close to her face.
- Get ready to have someone take pictures!

If She Gives Up

- Try a position change
- Remind her of the baby (have her touch the head, state the date of the baby's birthday, wonder what color the hair is, etc.)
- Sometimes another care provider can be helpful. Don't be afraid to enlist the nurse, doctor, or another family member for fresh encouragement.
- Point out all that she has accomplished so far. Praise her and let her know that you believe in her. Acknowledge her struggles, but don't give up on her.

Dan Townsend's words of wisdom for all those fathers out there:

"Don't get scared. Don't listen to horror stories and forget what you see on TV. You won't get all woozy from the sight of the blood, it really isn't that bad. Just get in there and persevere, you'll do fine and you won't mess it up...

Bible Study Discussion

1. Coaches, how do you feel about being able to support her during labor?

2. What have you done to practice?

3. Practice some of these techniques right now, finding out which ones she likes/dislikes.

4. How confident are you?

5. What part of this chapter stands out to you?

Part Two

Christ-Centered
Bible Study

They devoted themselves to the apostles' teaching and to the
fellowship, to the breaking of bread and to prayer.   Acts 2:42

Let me encourage you to take this Bible study and pray
that the Lord would send to you other couples who might be
interested in meeting every other week. You can gather for
prayer, the reading of scripture, eating together, and giving
support to one another as your families grow in the Lord.

Included in this section will be a basic topic outline. I pray
that your time together will be Spirit-led, with the group taking
time to hear from the Lord. Give yourselves 20 – 30 minutes at
the end of each session to just be quiet before God, and wait to
hear upon His voice. If any has a word of exhortation, if any
would like to sing in the Spirit, or if anyone has a need for prayer,
this is a good time to present these requests. Pray for the needs of
yourself or others, but be keen to saving time for prayer over
things that build up the Holy Spirit within your group.

Be still, and know that I am God
Psalm 46:10

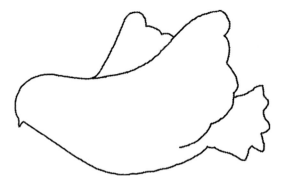

These weekly outlines are interchangeable, and a person can begin at any point within the Bible study. Appoint an elder over your group who fits the Titus 2 format, encouraging the men to fill that role, if possible. Pray that the Lord would send you someone who is skilled at guitar or keyboard who can lead you in 15-20 minutes of worship and hymns before you begin. Plan to spend at least two hours together, and add an hour if you choose to make it a potluck. Have fun, and grow daily in His grace!

What You Will Need: Holy Bible

Bible Study – Basic Guidelines

5:30pm – 6:30pm	*Potluck & Fellowship*
6:30pm – 6:50pm	*Worship*
6:50pm – 7:00pm	*Intro/Weekly happenings*
7:00pm – 7:30pm	*Elder reads appointed scripture & gives a short sermonette (Sermonette can be replaced by group participation if desired)*
7:30pm – 8:00pm	*Discussion questions (You can assign a topic about pregnancy and birth, having one or more read up on it and present the information at the next meeting)*
8:00pm – 8:30pm	*Spirit-led time before the Lord. Close with a worship song and prayer.*

Session One - Filled With Confidence

Pregnancy can be a fabulous time for the couple, but many keep hidden worries inside of them about work, finances, and the wherewithal to include another member into the family. Dedicate the next few weeks to resist worry and doubt. Pay attention to every time you have a negative thought and combat that thought with a prayer for someone's salvation, a worship song, and replace it with the positive alternative.

You must now assume not only a defensive posture against negative thoughts, but you must also wage war against any fearful arrow that pierces your soul. Pregnancy can be a time of confusion, discomfort, panic, inconvenience and frustration. Or, you can choose to only allow the positive and lovely aspects of pregnancy to saturate you as you joyfully experience the process of laboring for your loved one, as the Lord labored for you! Praise the Lord!

Assigned Scripture: Ephesians 6:10-20
Correlating Chapter: Armor of God

Discussion:

1. What has the Lord done recently to give you joy and peace during this pregnancy?

2. How has the enemy tried to infiltrate your mind to bring doubt and discouragement?

3. What things have you done to "build the temple" growing inside of you?

4. In what ways are you teaching your little one about the Lord. Song? Prayer? The touch of love?

5. How can the armor of God help you during this pregnancy?

Session Two – Seek Ye First

Sometimes it is easy to get caught up in the hullabaloo of life and not place our focus on the Lord. We strive and toil to fulfill the daily requirements, but miss that all-important quiet time in the morning with our Father. Let us remember that all the things we strive for will be added to us, if we first make Jesus Christ our priority.

Who of us can say that we haven't pushed our spiritual life aside to make room for a busy schedule, a deadline, or a time of much-sleep? "Sorry, God," we might say. "I just don't have time to go to church, things are falling apart at the office." Perhaps if we press in to the Lord as our first priority, the rest will be less chaotic. A popular saying says, "A Bible that is falling apart is usually read by someone who isn't." So true!

When we make Him our first priority, when we seek Him first before we turn to worldly counsel, when we make every effort to be in the will of God, knowing what that will might be because we have been seeking His face, then God promises that He will provide all that we need. Not all that we want; all that we need…

Assigned Scripture: John 6:25-34

Discussion:

1. In what ways are you spending time with the Lord?

2. Has the Lord made Himself known to you recently?

3. In what ways can we live out John 6:25-34 during pregnancy?

4. Do you have an immediate need right now?

5. Has God used you to help someone else? If yes, how so?

Session Three – Be Still

Take this session and devote it to hearing from the Lord. Pay extra close attention to the prompting of your heart to share with the group. Has the Lord placed something there that keeps surfacing? Now is the time to allow the Holy Spirit to flow through you and to the group. Even if there is no word of encouragement, let this be a time where you gather in His name and come before Him to sit at His feet. Be quiet before Him, and listen for His voice. Speak to the group those things that you hear.

What You Will Need: Holy Bible

Assigned Scripture: *Psalm 46*

Discussion:

Take this time and devote it entirely to the Lord. Be still before Him, and listen for His Spirit. After everyone has had a chance to quiet themselves, if you feel led, speak out about what God is prompting you to say. If there is a prayer need, speak it out, and let another pray over the situation. Close the session praying for the unborn. Petition the Lord to give you a new and intimate knowledge of this baby, and bring you into a very close relationship with him or her. At your ending prayer, join hands with the rest of the group in a circle and pray for strength and unity among all Christians. Pray that we will be united in Christ as one body that desires to glorify the Father in heaven!

Session Four – Reflecting His Love

God has encrypted His plan of love and salvation all throughout nature, and the human body is no exception. Tonight, make time to watch the video "A Child Is Born" by Zola Levitt.

What You Will Need:
A Child Is Born (Video) produced by Zola Levitt
www.levitt.com

Assigned Scripture: Leviticus 23
Correlating Chapter: Pregnancy: It's a God Thing

Discussion:

1. How do the feasts of Israel point to pregnancy?

2. What might the significance of these correlations be to us & the baby?

3. What are we going to do with this new information?

4. What are some other things in nature that point to Jesus Christ?

Session Five: Search Our Heart

The Father in Heaven is having a special relationship with your child at this very moment. He is mindful of every thought in the baby's mind, and all of the child's days are numbered according to God's will. As God knows this child, so we should seek to bond with him or her in as deep a way as possible. We connect with the baby on a physical level by interaction and touch, on an emotional level through expressions of love, and on a spiritual level through prayer and meditation. Devote tonight to your unborn baby, allowing yourself to fall in love with this child of God.

Assigned Scripture: Psalm 139

(Review the Worksheet: For The Love of Baby)

For the Love of Baby:
An Application for Birth

Love is patient, love is kind; love does not envy; love does not parade itself, is not puffed up; does not behave rudely, does not seek its own, is not provoked, thinks no evil; does not rejoice in iniquity, but rejoices in the truth; [7]*bears all things, believes all things, hopes all things, endures all things. Love never fails.*

List 3 examples of patience during birth: (*Love is patient)*

1.

2.

3.

List 3 kind things you can do for your baby during birth: (*love is kind)*

1.

2.

3.

List 3 consequences to comparing your birth with that of your friends/relatives. (*love does not envy)*

1.

2.

3.

List 3 benefits of privacy during birth: (*love does not parade itself*)

1.

2.

3.

List 3 prideful things that might hinder your progress in birth: (*is not puffed up*)

1.

2.

3.

List 3 rude behaviors by birthing women that you have heard about and how you will avoid them: (*does not behave rudely*)

1.

2.

3.

List 3 selfish things that a woman could do that might jeopardize the baby or the birth: (*does not seek its own*)

1.

2.

3.

List 3 possible things that could happen that go against your birth plan and how you might respond graciously to them. (*is not provoked*)

1.

2.

3.

List 3 positive thoughts to entertain during a contraction:
(*thinks no evil*)

1.

2.

3.

List 3 truths about normal childbirth that may be distorted by popular stories
(*does not rejoice in iniquity, but rejoices in the truth*)

1.

2.

3.

Explain why it is important to bear with the contractions in a way that does resist the efforts of the body, and give one example of how to do this: (*bears all things*)

List 3 truths about normal childbirth that you firmly believe: (*believes all things*)

1.

2.

3.

List 3 of your most important hopes for this birth: (*hopes all things*)

1.

2.

3.

Explain why enduring the work of childbirth is an act of love for your baby. (*endures all things*)

Explain why there are no failures in birth! (*Love never fails*)

NOTE: If during pregnancy it is found difficult to maintain these ideals, one can rest assured that Jesus Christ is able to fulfill all of these definitions of love, and He loves us unconditionally.

Session Six – Renew Your Mind

Birth is different from culture to culture. Women tend to conform to those around them when it comes to childbirth, having not much to go by when trying to get a mental picture of what it will be like. We rely on the accounts of family, friends, and the media to feed our imagination of what we can expect. However, this can be frightening to us and may give a foothold to Satan, allowing him to attack us with doubts and worries. Allow yourself to be transformed by the renewing of your mind, deleting all negative images of birth from your memory. Trust that God will give you exactly the birth that He has planned for you, and be ready to accept it with joy. Surrender to your Lord, trust in Him with all of your heart, and He will guide you.

What You Will Need:

Assigned Scripture: Romans 12
Correlating Chapter: The Natural Childbirth Tool Box

Discussion:

Discuss the following worksheet

Taking Every Thought Captive
Worksheet

Finally, brethren, whatsoever things are true, whatsoever things are
honest, whatsoever things are just, whatsoever things are pure,
whatsoever things are lovely, whatsoever things are of good report; if
there be any virtue, and if there be any praise, think on these things.
Philippians 4:8

1. Things about birth that are true:
   (*whatsoever things are true*)

2. Birthing myths:

3. Being honest, I feel this way about birth:
   (*whatsoever things are honest*)

4. Ways that my care providers can be honest:

5. Ways that my care proveders may be dishonest:

6. My rights as a birthing mother:
   (*whatsoever things are just*)

7. What should be expected from me as a birthing mother:

8. I describe a pure birth as:
   (*whatsoever things are pure*)

9. Things that could cause my birth to be less than pure:

10. The most lovely things about birth are:
   (*whatsoever things are lovely*)

11. Things about birth that may be difficult, yet still lovely:

12. A positive birth story that someone told me:
   (*whatsoever things are of good report*)

13. What are the virtues of birth (example - patience):
   (*if there be any virtue*)

14. If you were to praise a woman on her birth experience, what kinds of things would you praise her for?:
(*and if there be any praise*)

Think on these things…

Session Seven – Lay It Down

Anxiety. It can creep up and plague you at any point in your pregnancy or birth. You have perfected the putting on of the spiritual armor each day, yet although you are prepared, the anxiety still has a way of coming. That which holds you, you must let go of. Lay it down at the feet of the Lord, and trust in Him to take care of it. The act of surrendering to Him is the sweetest freedom one can ever experience. Now is the time, don't wait a moment longer. Loosen the grip of your hand from around your situation and place every corner of your heart's trust into His hands. You will be blessed!

Assigned Scripture: Philippians 4
Correlating Chapter: Fear Not

Discussion:

1. Practice Abdominal Breathing

2. Try out different positions for labor

3. Try out different positions for delivery

4. Discuss any fears you might be having (Dads too!)

5. How can fear be affecting the decisions being made by women during birth?

6. What are some of the consequences of those decisions made from fear?

7. What are some measures you will be taking to help reduce fear and facilitate security at the birth site?

Session Eight – A New Beginning

Your baby is almost here! Are you ready? Life changes in marvelous ways and God is right there with us as it happens. He is faithful to us and never leaves us. With a Godly confidence, forge ahead with the power of the Holy Spirit to fulfill the perfect will of the Lord. Let everything that comes about be used for the furtherance of the gospel, so that Christ might be preached in not only your words, but your actions as well.

Assigned Scripture: Philippians 1
Correlating Chapter: Coaching Techniques

Discussion:

1. How has your pregnancy/birth been a testimony to Christ Jesus so far?

2. In what way would you like to bring glory to the Lord through this experience?

3. Have you had opportunity to witness to a non-believer about your faith in Christ as it relates to this experience?

4. How will the birth attendants know that you are Christian?

5. As you part ways, would you like to continue in fellowship with each other? If yes, then how so? Bible study? More potlucks?

Birth Testimony Encore

I believe in divine coincidence. The day I was preparing to send this book to the printer, I received an email with the following three birth testimonies attached. After reading them, I was convinced that I should include them here for you to read.

As you read them you will feel encouraged, be empowered, become concerned, have your spirit lifted, shed a tear or two, and rejoice over the wonderful way God takes any situation and uses it for His good will and purpose. Stacy's life was changed through her births. I would hope that God's intention for that goes beyond her life and extends to yours as well.

Our Birth Stories

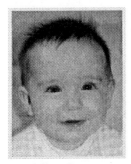 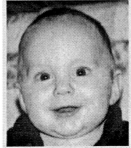 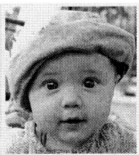

Madeline Grace   Zachary Luke   Chloe Faith

Our story begins the first week of August 1997. I was suspicious that I was pregnant and had taken a pregnancy test. As I held my breath in anticipation, I was in such disbelief when the test was positive. We had been told that due to my history of endometriosis that we would most likely have a difficult time getting pregnant or would need some medical assistance to achieve a pregnancy. I immediately went into our bedroom to awaken my husband, Todd and tell him the news. He was working nights and was sleeping at that time of the afternoon. I informed him that "The test . . .It has two lines. . .It has two lines!" He wasn't awake enough to process the information at first, but soon came out of the bedroom in disbelief to verify what I was telling him. He wasn't aware that I thought I might be pregnant or had even purchased a test. We were so excited! In fact, we were so excited that I took 4 tests – just for the fun of watching them all turn positive. We wanted to wait a while to tell our family, but our excitement overtook us and we told them the very next day.

I started calling that afternoon to see which OB/GYN doctor I could see. We had only been in town a month at that point, and I was, thus, classified as a 'new patient'. Therefore, I only found one doctor who had an opening before my 16th week of pregnancy. This being my first pregnancy, I of course, thought I had to see a physician right away. I went into my first appointment at 10 weeks gestation. Todd and I heard the heartbeat for the first time and I couldn't help but giggle in amazement.

As the pregnancy progressed, I began to feel rushed and hurried through my appointments with this physician. I attributed it to my being an anxious, first time mom and figured it was just the way things were run in a busy obstetrical office. I became even more disillusioned with this physician when I called during my 36th week of pregnancy with a question regarding pain. My legs had been bothering me enough that I was consistently missing work and needing Tylenol around the clock just to function in my daily activities. I was told that no one was comfortable during her last trimester of pregnancy and to just "deal with it." They did not think I needed to be seen or treated so I thought I was probably over-reacting and the leg pains must be a normal part of pregnancy. We later found out that my leg pains were due to a chronic health condition.

To prepare for the upcoming birth, we took a weekend childbirth class. Even though it was interesting and fun, we did not feel we learned much new information. I had just graduated from nursing school, and had a wonderful obstetrical rotation where I saw many unassisted and un-medicated births. I subconsciously assumed that my childbirth experience would go that way. Todd and I felt we knew everything we needed to know in order to have the birth experience we dreamed about. We knew that childbirth could be unpredictable, but we could not have guessed all we would experience while having our babies through the upcoming years.

On April 1, 1998 at 1:00 a.m., I was awakened from a deep sleep by my bag of waters breaking. We excitedly called the doctor and went into the hospital. Labor still had not started by 7:00 that morning, so it was decided to start a pitocin drip. Then our 'perfect delivery' started to deteriorate. The contractions quickly grew very strong and intense. I tried to relax, focus, and breathe like they had taught us in class; however, I found those techniques to be aggravating, irritating, and ineffective. I was therefore left with no other coping mechanisms. Even small insignificant things were impossible for me to deal with. Todd was trying so hard to help me to relax and to be supportive, but he had just had lunch and the smell of BBQ chicken on his breath was more than I could effectively handle. I was not very pleasant to him at that point.

The pitocin was titrated to a point where I wasn't getting much of a break between strong contractions. They were unrelenting. I was crying, tensing up, scared, and fighting what my body was trying to do with all I was worth. I was in such fear of the pain of the next painful contraction and how much longer I would be able to endure the discomfort, that I couldn't effectively work with the pain of the present contraction. It became an unproductive cycle that only increased my overall fear, pain, and panicked state of mind. I was given some narcotics to help, but I did not find them very effective. In addition, I had a low-grade fever, stomach cramps, vomiting and diarrhea. It was later determined that I had a stomach virus in addition to the discomforts of giving birth.

After five hours, my cervix was checked and I had only dilated to 2 cm. I was so devastated and scared. It seemed almost more than I could endure. How was I going to go on? After all of this pain and discomfort, I had only come that far? Afterward, my mother told me that I repeatedly asked her, in all honesty, if I was dying. I knew at that point I was beat, and requested an epidural. Once it was placed, I fell into a deep sleep and awakened fully dilated and ready to push. At this point I remember thinking, "At least I didn't need a C-section!"

At first, I couldn't feel my muscles enough to push and was ineffective in my efforts, so the medication in the epidural was reduced. I continued to have stomach cramps that hurt as much as the contractions accompanied with more vomiting and diarrhea. After three hours of pushing with no progress, I was exhausted. The physician told me that it was time to have a C-section. The baby's head was not engaging in my pelvis correctly. My heart just fell. I truly was not going to have the perfect birth I wanted. To add to my disappointment, the doctor told me I 'earned' my C-section and I therefore, perceived that I was a failure. In hindsight, I think she said I was a 'failure to progress,' a medical term – but I heard and remembered 'failure.'

It was with a heavy heart that I was wheeled to the operating room. However, I was so exhausted that there was a part of me that was glad to finally see my baby – even if the road led us here. They gave me more oral medications, which I promptly vomited all over Todd's hand

and arm, and restarted the epidural. I remember being strapped down and feeling them tug and pull on my abdomen. What a strange feeling! When they said the baby was out, I remember thinking: "Please be a girl . . . please be a girl . . ."

"It's a girl!" they announced. Madeline Grace was here! A healthy baby girl weighing 7 lbs, 5 oz. It was 8:00 pm. The first pictures we have of her are as they were lifting her out of my abdomen. She had her arms uplifted ready to embrace the world. I heard her first little cry and it did not even register with me that it was my baby. It was a small, tiny cry because all the medications given to me were affecting her. Todd left my side to go see her. He brought her over to me with tears in his eyes and I took my first look at her. I saw her little 'angel kisses' (stork bites) on her nose and that was the last thing I remember- I fell into a deep sleep.

Upon awakening an hour later, cold and shivering uncontrollably in a dark corner of the recovery room, I overheard the nurses and doctors discussing a case in which multiple units of blood had been given to a mother for a hemorrhage. I was terrified they were talking about me.

A nurse finally came over and assured me that I didn't need a blood transfusion and that my baby was doing fine in the nursery. Todd soon came up to the recovery room from the nursery and informed me that Maddie had my toes; short and stubby. What a funny thing to notice!

From that point on I really don't remember much – I held her for the first time and talked with my family and friends, but I don't remember any of it. If we didn't have pictures of the events, I wouldn't have known they occurred.

Slowly the realization of the loss of the birth experience I had wanted began to make its impact on me. I cried often and felt depressed, although I couldn't have named it as such at the time. I felt like a horrible mother who was a failure at her first major task of motherhood. Upon leaving the hospital, I could hardly walk down the hallway of the Birth Center without crying – I wanted Maddie back inside of me, so I could do the labor again and 'do it better.' I thought I had deserved my C-section because I was a terrible patient who couldn't handle labor like most women could. However, I did realize I was so blessed to have had a healthy baby girl.

At the urging of a friend who had been in Nursing a long time, I ordered my hospital records and learned that my diagnosis was

Cephalopelvic Disproportion (CPD) - where the baby's head won't fit through the mother's pelvis. The physician verbally told us that Maddie had cocked her head and was thus in a malposition, however, it was never documented in my records. The delivering pediatrician said that her head was not in an incorrect position, but that she did have quite a 'cone head' from being in the birth canal so long.

I continued to have Post-Partum difficulties. I split open my incision getting into the car leaving the hospital, which developed into a mild infection. I also developed a uterine infection resulting from a torn cervix that took months to resolve. The delivering physician was not appropriately aggressive in treating me and allowed the infection to continue. The pain and fevers only added to my physical pain and discomfort. I realized this could have been an easily avoidable situation.

At my 6-week Post-Partum check-up, I was not thoroughly examined after having the infection even though I was still complaining of some symptoms. I had become very frustrated with this doctor and I decided I needed to go to my family physician for a physical. He discovered a significant yeast infection that was not diagnosed and strongly urged me to see another OB/GYN to determine if the uterine infection had resolved. I returned to a previous doctor in another city who had treated me in the past. He immediately had me scheduled for surgery. He was concerned the infection had spread from my uterus, out through my fallopian tubes and into my pelvic region. I had a laproscopy and D & C (dilation and curettage). They did discover a chronically infected uterus, as well as a large ovarian cyst, and treated me with IV antibiotics overnight in the hospital and a round of oral medications at home

As I look back on this experience, I can see where Post Partum Depression affected me, as well as the drain on my physical health from all the post-delivery complications. I was so jealous when I heard other women tell of their birth stories in which things had gone the way they wanted. I would even cry if I saw a 'normal' birth on a television program. My leg and arm pain became more pronounced and I was later diagnosed with fibromyalgia. Its onset was most likely exacerbated by my childbirth experience and complicated recovery.

Looking back, I honestly think the C-section could have most likely been avoided had I known about and utilized some common sense mechanics of childbirth. God designed a woman's body beautifully to give birth. For example, a few techniques include staying mobile and active throughout labor and delivery, relaxation, proper breathing, and avoiding an epidural. All these would have helped my body to labor efficiently, just like it was designed and created.

However, even though this experience was difficult, I was amazed at how much I loved that little baby. I loved her big blue eyes, her baby sounds, her brown hair that continuously stood on end, and her giggles. She was the joy of my life. She brought such joy and light into our house. I would go through the whole experience again if it meant I would have her. If given the choice, however, I would choose to go about things differently with my next delivery.

When we decided to expand our family, it took us almost a year to conceive and for our pregnancy test to 'have two lines'. The concern had been that the chronic uterine infection had affected my fallopian tubes. Once we conceived, I chose a new doctor who had come highly recommended from several friends and acquaintances. I really wanted to deliver this baby vaginally. I so mourned the loss of the 'normal' experience the first time around and wanted to do whatever I could to maximize my chances of having a VBAC (Vaginal Birth after Cesarean).

I asked a friend who had two natural, un-medicated births how she did it. It seemed like such an unattainable goal and something I could not understand anyone being able to do. She told me she and her husband took a 12 - week natural childbirth class and that it would be worth looking into. I researched it and thought that it would be the road for us to investigate and travel down. What appealed to me was how it taught a woman to work with her body, with the help of a coach, so she didn't fight the contractions and halt/complicate her labor progress.

I asked the physician what he thought my chances were of having a VBAC. I felt he was supportive at first – told me I had about a 50/50 chance of delivering vaginally, but to give it a try. As time went on, I began to feel that we had different perspectives on the situation – I saw the glass as half full and he saw it as half empty. He said the natural childbirth classes or any childbirth coping techniques wouldn't be of any benefit to us since I was looking at a 'square peg/round hole' scenario in relation to my pelvis outlet and the baby's head. In his opinion, I would more than likely have another C-section anyway.

I asked Todd to accompany me to my next appointment to make sure I was hearing the doctor right and was processing what he was telling me correctly. I was concerned I wasn't hearing what I wanted to hear, and was therefore, not being realistic about the situation. If I truly needed a C-section, then I would gladly do it. However, with a 50/50 chance of avoiding one, I didn't want to undergo that major surgery if I didn't have to.

I was concerned that I was being a difficult patient and was expecting too much from my physician. Why else would I have had trouble with two doctors? Was it me? Did I need to stop asking questions? Were my expectations too high? Did I just need to have a scheduled C-section? Was I putting my baby boy at an unnecessary risk by wanting to take the unknown outcome of labor versus the relative known safety of a scheduled C-section? My ultimate goal was 'Healthy mom - healthy baby," but I knew that if I didn't at least give a VBAC delivery an honest try, I would regret it for the rest of my life.

At this particular appointment, I concluded that this doctor was not the one we wanted or needed for this delivery. He rushed me through that appointment, was upset that Maddie was present, and was short mannered with us. He told me he had many more patients to see that day and he did not have time to answer my questions. He had me lie down on the table so he could measure my uterus while I asked questions - to save time. In the process, he tripped over Maddie, which made her cry, and caused him to become irritated. The appointment continued to go downhill from there.

I asked what I thought was a very pertinent question: since I had fibromyalgia and my muscles tended to tire and fatigue easily and quickly, would he and/or the nurses monitor me more closely and how long would he let me labor before he would intervene? He replied with "Are you implying that I don't watch my patients and don't provide good care?" Of course, that was not what I was implying and I burst into tears. He stood up to leave, and told us he didn't have the time for us anymore, as we were the cause of making him late for his many other patients he had to see the afternoon. The whole appointment was maybe 20 minutes in length. We left with the decision that it would be in my best interest to have the C-section during the 38th week of pregnancy so I would not inconvenience anyone by going into labor during the physician's off hours.

I was so upset that I literally wept and sobbed off and on for three days. All I wanted was a chance and for someone to support me in my 50% chance of being successful. I called and discussed the situation with my childbirth instructor through tears. She suggested I contact a Certified Nurse Midwife here in town who delivers babies in the hospital. Her husband is an OB/GYN physician and they are in practice together – he as her medical/surgical back-up.

Todd and I went in to see her at 30 weeks of pregnancy with two pages of questions! She was so encouraging that I knew instantly that she was the one we needed to deliver our baby. Upon informing the previous doctor we were changing providers, he became fairly defensive and unpleasant. He implied that we were making an unwise decision. Nevertheless, after much prayer, we were certain we were making the right decision and were looking forward to the upcoming birth.

At our first appointment with the midwife, she immediately pointed out things that had gone wrong in our first labor that could most likely be avoided during this upcoming labor. Examples that come to mind are taking antibiotics to prevent my water from breaking prematurely, avoiding an epidural so I could be mobile and help the baby position correctly in my pelvis, and not having pitocin. She was very thorough and provided an extensive physical exam and a pelvimetry. It was her opinion that before we decided to try a vaginal birth, we should probably measure my pelvic outlet and see if there was adequate room for the baby to pass. It was her clinical determination that there was sufficient space for a baby.

We felt like we had a game plan and a birth plan we with which were comfortable. If we wanted to try a VBAC, she was behind us and supportive of our efforts. If we had problems in the delivery and needed a C-section, the physician would be in the hospital ready to perform the surgery. Maddie enjoyed accompanying me to my remaining appointments and developed a special relationship with the midwife.

In the meantime, we were attending natural childbirth classes and learning how to labor effectively. We practiced relaxation techniques, daily exercises and stretches, and focused on eating a high protein diet. Todd would put clothespins on various parts of my body to simulate contractions. They hurt, but were a great way to practice relaxation. We felt we learned a great deal and were more prepared for this delivery. We had many 'tricks in our bag'. In case one coping technique didn't work, we had another one to try.

On July 17, 2001 at 11:45 p.m. I was once again awakened from a deep sleep by my water breaking. Ironically, Todd had just finished packing his bags for the hospital thinking we had 3 weeks left. He had just turned off 'The Late Show with David Letterman" and was in the process of turning out the bedroom lights. I was 37 weeks pregnant – 3 weeks early. How could this happen again? This labor was starting exactly the same way as the first one! We had been trying hard to prevent this. I knew I needed the amniotic fluid to help the baby position correctly. I lay back on the bed and cried. Eventually we knew it was time and we had no choice but to call the midwife, our parents, Jocelyn, (our friend who was our co-coach – she had had 3 VBAC'S and was pregnant with her 5th baby at the time), and a neighbor to come and stay with Maddie.

When we arrived at the hospital parking garage, we took a moment to pray. We knew the situation was not in our control and asked for God's direction, assistance, and guidance. We prayed the prayer that never fails – "Lord, Your will be done." We then went to the hospital with the attitude that we had a job to do and we were going to give it everything we had. With that, we grabbed our bags and headed off to the Emergency Department entrance.

An orderly came to wheel me up to the Birth Center. The tears started again. I was so apprehensive and anxious. How would this labor turn out? Would I be disappointed if things didn't go as I wanted? Would I struggle with feelings of being a failure and deal with depression again? Would I be able to cope with the pain without an epidural or other pain medication?

Upon being admitted, they started an IV, drew routine blood work and applied the external fetal monitor. These were prerequisites for having a VBAC. They wanted to carefully monitor for the rare, but very real risk of uterine rupture. A physical exam showed that I was 4 cm dilated with no active labor pattern. That was much further than we had gotten the first time before I had an epidural after hours of ineffective labor. That was a good sign indeed. However the baby was at a –3 station, which was too high in my pelvis. He was also "sunny side up" (posterior) – meaning he was looking at my stomach versus my spine. It doesn't make vaginal deliveries impossible, just more difficult.

We tried to rest and 2 hours later, I had dilated to 6 cm with little or no contractions, yet the baby had not descended down beyond a –3 station. The odds were now starting to rise against us. It was decided that some pitocin was needed to stimulate a more active labor pattern and bring the baby down. I was very leery of the drug since it seemed to be such a significant part of the equation with my first birth. They gave it to me slowly and increased it by only 2 mU at a time instead of doubling the dose at each increase.

At this point I remember looking over at Todd and Jocelyn and realized how tired I was. I just wanted to curl up and take a nap. Todd put on Maddie's "Sleep Sound In Jesus" CD by Michael Card, which is such a comforting lullaby album, and we all settled in for a nap; Todd on the cot, Jocelyn in the rocking chair, and me in the cozy bed.

I could feel the contractions starting to grow in frequency and intensity, but was so relaxed they did not bother me. I could hear people talking but was too tired and relaxed to respond. I was not very alert or aware of my surroundings. This rest and sleep was probably what helped to give me the physical strength I needed to continue throughout the entire labor.

Two and a half hours later, I suddenly woke with a full bladder. On the way to the bathroom, the contractions came on with great intensity. The best description I can give is that they felt like very painful menstrual cramps in combination with strong gas pains. They started low in my abdomen, moved upward and then moved back down. It took a conscious effort with each one to relax. My body wanted to automatically tense up. I could hear Todd, the midwife, and Jocelyn notice parts of my body that were tense and needed to be relaxed - mainly my shoulders, forehead and legs. Once I noticed and made an effort to relax even those small body parts, the pain greatly subsided. Singing songs in my head from church worship services helped to calm me emotionally and spiritually so I was able to focus on relaxing physically.

I was also comforted to know that the physician was in the hospital. He came by to check on us a few times. If my uterus ruptured or if I needed an emergency C-section for any reason, he was there and ready to operate.

The contractions continued to gain in intensity and frequency. I was at 8 cm already! This was where natural childbirth training was invaluable to us. I had coping mechanisms and tools to help me relax and concentrate in order to get through labor, one contraction at a time. It was a choice with each one – am I going to do what I need to do to relax my way through this contraction or am I going to tense up and fight it? I took it one contraction at a time. I knew if I started to worry about how long labor was going to last or how painful it was going to get, I would lose my perspective and therefore lose control. The more tense I was, the more painful the contractions became. I had intense pain in my lower uterus and I was sure that my uterus was rupturing. No one else seemed concerned, so I assumed I was okay. The pitocin was then turned off which helped.

Soon I felt on overwhelming desire to push – intense pressure. I pushed for over an hour since the baby was having a hard time navigating his way under my pubic bone. The midwife had me push and labor in many positions – lying on my side, standing, squatting, kneeling, and hanging off the edge of the bed and on the toilet. I felt like I was not making any progress and that I did not have much control over the situation. It was a surreal experience. My body had taken over. I made so many moaning, growling and other noises that my throat was sore for days afterwards. I had broken capillaries on my face and shoulders that lasted for days as well. Todd said I prayed out loud for God's help consistently throughout the day. I have no recollection of that, but it evidently helped.

The midwife eventually said she could see the head and I honestly thought she was lying to me. I had heard that many times the first time around with Maddie's birth – and I thought she wanted to give me a reason to keep going even though I wasn't making much progress. She told me to reach down and feel his head. It didn't register with me that I was actually feeling my baby's head – he was coming! She said one more push and we'd be there. I still had my doubts. Until the baby started to crown. That was incredibly painful and it burned intensely. The next push was even worse. That was probably the worst part of the labor. If I was one to swear, I'm sure there would have been many words spoken that point. I felt I was ripping apart. Amazingly, I did not need an episiotomy and did not have any perineal tearing.

I heard, "The head's out!" the burning let up and I looked down and could see his little head between my legs. Unbelievable! So this is what it is like! My first thoughts were "We did it!" He had turned around from the posterior position at just the right time. The midwife told me to reach down and pull him out – I was too tired to pull him all the way onto my chest, but I did pull him out onto my belly. He was so warm and slippery and had that so sweet newborn smell. Here was Zachary Luke at a healthy 6 lbs, 13 oz, born at 12:56 pm on July 18.

They soon took him over to the warmer and I was relieved to hear him cry. In the meantime, I was delivering the placenta. That was uncomfortable and I was glad to have it out. I felt empty then, but it was a good, 'full' feeling of empty. The nurses continued with painful uterine massages and the resulting blood clots were large and painful to pass.

I tried to breastfeed Zachary, but he was only interested in nuzzling. I didn't mind because it gave me an opportunity to look at him. He looked so different than my little Maddie did. He had a slimmer face, a sharper chin, less hair and his feet and hands were so blue, but he was beautiful to me.

The midwife came over and gave me a hug. I overheard her tell Todd and Jocelyn that I came into the office just asking for a chance, and look what I just did. She leaned over and told me that I should call my previous doctor and tell him the outcome. I thought she was kidding, but upon questioning her later, discovered she was serious. There would be another woman in my situation that would come through his door some day and he should know that there is hope for everyone. A few weeks later, I did call his office to relay the news of our successful VBAC. I had to leave a message with his nurse and never heard back from him.

I was still in disbelief at that point. It was one of the hardest things I had ever done. Maddie's birth was hard in its duration, complications, exhaustion, undergoing major surgery and depression. Zachary's was hard in that I had pitocin. But with no pain medication, I felt every contraction and move he made on his way out. Since we were better prepared for the delivery and effectively used the techniques we learned in childbirth class, I never felt the pain was unmanageable or unbearable and did not come to the point of wanting/needing medications.

Forty-five minutes after I delivered, I was placed in a wheel chair and was on my way to my postpartum room. As Zachary was placed in my lap and we were moving through the hospital, I kept thinking, "Wow, we did it! Thank you, Lord!" We were off to meet all his grandparents, Aunt Stephanie and big sister, Maddie, of course.

The feelings I had were feelings of validation, amazement, gratefulness, success, happiness, pride, and femininity. Until that moment, I had always mourned the loss of those feelings with the first experience.

Upon discharge from the hospital, our midwife filled us in on what had transpired. Even though I had adequate room in my pelvis, it was shaped more like a male's than a female's (an android pelvis). After conferring with the doctor, she did not think it would be an issue and did not tell me. I was glad I didn't know that until after I delivered. I would probably have just scheduled the C-section. She also told us that she wasn't going to tell me when to push. She wanted my body to work on it's own. She didn't want me to push prematurely and risk settling the baby's head at the wrong angle. She mentioned she was glad we came to her with the attitude that we were not entitled to a VBAC, had done our research, were open to a C-section if it was necessary, and just wanted a chance to try. She told me I was an inspiration to VBAC's everywhere and should consider speaking at VBAC classes in the community.

She said we gave her a few gray hairs, but overcame many odds. The first being a diagnosis of CPD, an android shaped pelvis,

Bacterial Vaginosis (which played a part in my water breaking by making the bag of water less pliable), ruptured bag of waters, baby at a high station and posterior position, the use of pitocin, an early delivery, no spontaneous active labor pattern, and a previous C-section.

I often wonder if God in His wisdom had my labor start at 37 weeks for a reason, even if it seemed like a negative occurrence to us. If I had gone into labor closer to my due date, I wonder if I might not have been able to have a VBAC delivery. Zachary was a big baby for 37 weeks, and who knew how much bigger he would have been with 3 more weeks of growth in the womb.

Our successful outcome was due to our brilliant and caring Health Care Providers, our childbirth educator, and most of all from God's grace and His assistance. He heard and answered our prayers for a natural and un-medicated delivery. It will be fun to see how our next delivery goes if He decides to gift us with another baby.

In June 2003, we discovered that God had indeed blessed us with another baby. Baby number three was due in February 2004. My pregnancy was uncomplicated with the exception of Fibromyalgia (FM) symptoms that interfered with my daily routines and emotions, but nothing that was a true obstetrical concern. I tried to cherish the special moments and fetal movements since this was more than likely my last pregnancy.

We planned on having a family birth with Madeline and Zachary present to witness the birth and the plans for preparing the children began in earnest. We watched childbirth videos, read books, and attended classes and tours of the Birth Center at the hospital. Maddie was especially excited about the upcoming birth of her little sister since she had been praying for one for a while.

I was more anxious about when this labor would start than with the previous ones since there were more logistical things that needed attention. For example, who would watch the kids, who would get Maddie to school, when did the kids need to get to the hospital and who would be with them, the weather, etc. I had prayed often for God's ultimate timing and coordination with this birth.

At 39 weeks gestation, I had about 36 hours of a gastrointestinal upset with diarrhea and cramps. I went to bed around 11:00 pm on February 14 and was awakened at 2:00 am with more cramping and diarrhea, however this time the diarrhea had become bloody. I was now concerned that there was something significantly wrong with my gastrointestinal (GI) tract. Especially since I had Irritable Bowel

Syndrome (IBS), which can often flare up and cause a variety of problems for me. IBS is often associated with FM and GI upsets were just a normal part of life for me. I wondered in the back of my mind if perhaps I had started labor, especially since I lost my mucous plug that night. The pains were not coming very consistently and my uterus remained soft. The pain was mostly located in my lower left abdomen and each spasm was accompanied with loose, bloody stools. With this information, I determined that I was most likely not in labor.

At 4:00 am, the pain and bleeding had increased so I awakened Todd and told him I needed some help. Knowing that before we called anyone or went to the hospital, they would want to know if I had contacted my Obstetrical provider. Therefore, we decided to call our Certified Nurse Midwife first. Since it did not seem like a typical labor pattern and knowing my medical history, she suggested taking an anti-diarrhea medication first and to be in contact with her again soon.

I tried to lie down and relax through the pain thinking that if relaxation worked so well in the past for labor contractions, maybe it could be of help for intestinal spasms. After about 2 or 3 intestinal spasms, I had intense pain in my lower abdomen that had me sitting straight up in bed unable to move and out of breath. What was happening? These pains/spasms were definitely not like anything I had ever experienced before. The diarrhea and rectal bleeding increased despite the anti-diarrhea medication. At this point, I became scared that something was significantly wrong with my GI system. Again, I ran through my mental checklist to see if labor had started, but the pain was irregular and located mostly in my lower left abdomen again and my uterus remained soft. I had Todd feel my abdomen during a spasm to verify my assessment.

Our midwife, at this point, had us call my gastroenterologist who told us to come to the Emergency Department and he would meet us down there. Todd called for our friend Nicole to come and stay with the kids and then loaded the car with our belongings. He thought that since we were 39 weeks pregnant it might not be a bad idea to pack all our belongings for labor.

In the meantime, I was in incredible pain. I was so scared and was crying, groaning, and actually yelling for help. Nicole called her husband and asked him to call the people in our church small group to pray for us since I was obviously very ill. I could not remain still and was pacing around the bedroom and bathroom. Ironically, I remember telling Todd, quite loudly, that this was so much worse than labor! In hindsight, had I known I was having contractions, I honesty think I could have handled the pain better. I knew how to relax and contractions were something that was familiar to me. I knew what caused the pain, that it was not due to a health problem or emergency, and I knew how to work with them. I knew that contractions, though not a pleasant experience, were a normal process that would bring me the incredible gift of our baby.

These pains did not feel like any contraction I had ever had before. It is a great example of how fear can cause increased and unnecessary pain in childbirth. I wondered if they would want to do a C-section at the hospital to be able to treat whatever type of GI infections/disturbance/colitis I may have had.

I was standing at the bathroom sink waiting for Todd to come and get me for the ride to the hospital. I was wondering how I was going to endure the car ride, the pain was so intense. I was concerned that if I did not get this under control, I would not be able to handle labor when it started –especially if this triggered labor. I knew I needed medical attention and I had to go, but seriously wondered how I was going to do it. I reminded myself that people every day in serious, if not more intense pain, make the trip to the hospital and it was something I was just going to have to do. I was too scared to make the drive to the hospital and too scared to stay home as well. What a dilemma. I was convinced something was definitely wrong.

Nicole came in to give me my coat and I remember telling her through tears that this was awful and I was not even having contractions. By the time Todd got there, I was bent over the sink, legs locked and couldn't move. He told me it was time to get into the car. I snapped at him and responded with 'Don't talk to me! I can't move and I'm not going anywhere! I'm not getting in the car – I just can't do it!" He said, "Okay, then I'm calling 911". At this point, he had clued into the fact that I was acting and sounding like I was in the transition part of labor, but dismissed the idea because I told him I was not in labor and wasn't having contractions (at least having contractions like I thought I should be having contractions).

I knew something significant was occurring if I was glad for an ambulance. That is something I would normally choose not to do unless it was definitely indicated since that is a drastic step to take. However, I have to admit that one of my first reactions was relief. I was thinking that they could give me some pain medication for the intestinal cramps much sooner than I could get it if I was in the Emergency Department. I wanted to get the pain under control so I could effectively handle labor contractions when I went into labor. I was worried that this additional stress on my body would put me into labor soon.

He ran downstairs to call the paramedics and I made my way over to the bed and was leaning over the side yelling to him "something was wrong." I was thinking in terms of gastrointestinal problems though, not an impending birth. I was praying and pleading for God's help and guidance.

While on the phone with the dispatcher, they timed my pains and they were 1 minute apart. He removed my sweat pants to see if any part of the baby was emerging. There were no body parts, but there was a lot of bloody vaginal show and a bulging perineum. At this point, he knew birth was imminent. Since I was so upset, scared, and sure something was wrong, he didn't know if I was going to deliver a dead baby or a live baby, but a baby was coming for sure. I could hear the adrenaline, excitement, and tension in his voice as he said "Looks like the baby is coming!"

"No way" was my first thought – "I am not in labor! I'm not having a baby at home in our bed!"

He laid me down onto the bed just as the neighborhood firefighters were coming up the stairs. Paramedics arrived moments later. I felt the pelvic floor pressure and realized subconsciously that I was having a baby, but I was in denial thinking that if I did not push, I wasn't going to deliver there in our bed.

I looked over and saw Maddie standing by my bed. I had awakened her with my loud vocalizations. She was pale and was looking at me with scared, big eyes. Todd assured her the firefighters and ambulance personnel were there to help 'Mommy have her baby." One of the firefighters moved her toward Nicole and she took her downstairs. I prayed for her knowing how scared she was. I wanted her at the birth, but couldn't find the strength to request to have her there. I wasn't thinking too clearly or logically. She told us later that her legs were shaking due to fear, but Nicole reminded her about all we had talked about with having babies and she calmed down. Even though we planned on a family birth, her reaction surprised me. I think if we had worked into labor slowly, she would have responded better. Having all this happen in her home during the night was not something we had talked about or prepared her for.

I was flat on my back and really wanted to sit more upright, so Todd got behind me to support me, and a firefighter was there to catch the baby. I was still in disbelief and told Todd that I was not having a baby. He responded with "Yes, you are – the head is half way out – feel the baby, Stace!" I reached down and sure enough, there was a head there!

"Oh man, I remember this burning feeling – I am giving birth!" I suddenly realized. At this point, I made the mental transition over from having a GI disturbance and being ill to delivering a baby. I pulled my legs back and pushed again. I could feel the rest of her head emerging and Todd saying, "Wow, the head is out!" I pushed again and could feel the shoulders emerge, but I was still uncomfortable. One more push and the baby was out. It was 6:10 am Sunday, February 15, 2004. Little Chloe Faith was here! So there really was a baby in there! Could this little baby really be the one that was inside me for 39 weeks? What a miraculous thing.

The fireman caught her in a towel and I looked down in total disbelief at her little body. Todd announced that is was indeed a girl. She was covered in vernix. She then cried and they let me hold her for a minute while Maddie, Zachary, and Nicole came upstairs to see her. What a relief that she was healthy and crying lustily. She had "angel kisses' on her left eyebrow and a fair amount of brown hair. She looked somewhat like Maddie did upon her birth, but with lighter hair. The whole experience felt surreal and I kept thinking that it was unbelievable that I delivered in our bed. My bedding was soaked with blood and amniotic fluid but the firemen and paramedics, thankfully, saved our mattress and carpeting by using every towel they could find in our bathroom.

The kids came upstairs and crawled up onto my bed by my head and looked at her. Maddie said "She's so cute" and Zachary just continued to look at her. He was more interested in the firemen and fire truck than the baby. Nicole then took them back downstairs so I could finish delivering the placenta and the paramedics could check the baby. A fireman held her in the rocking chair in our room and administered oxygen to her – as a precaution, but she was doing fine.

I was having intense afterbirth pains, but the placenta did not deliver, so after 45 minutes, it was time to go to the hospital. I tried to walk down the stairs, but was a little dizzy, so they put me in a sling seat and carried me downstairs, strapped me onto a gurney and then wheeled me out to the waiting ambulance. How embarrassing - early on a Sunday morning and there was a fire truck and an ambulance in front of our house. How much more commotion could I make in our neighborhood on a quiet Sunday morning? I had on only my shirt, socks, and underwear, but was covered in a blanket. Todd was dressed, but didn't have his shoes on – only his slippers. We didn't even have our cameras.

The ride in the ambulance was uncomfortable due to the retained placenta and intense afterbirth pains. I knew they got worse with each baby, and that was definitely true for me. Todd rode up front with the paramedic and another fireman was back with me holding the baby. It was a long ride, but I remember the incredible sunrise upon leaving the house and how pretty the mountains looked.

When we arrived in the Emergency Department, I was embarrassed again to be wheeled in front of a full and busy department. They took me up to the Birth Center where it seemed like hundreds of nurses embarked upon us – some for Chloe and some for me.

The nurses at the Birth Center of the hospital delivered the placenta with no complications and then weighed and measured the baby. She was 7 pounds 8 ounces and 20 inches long. My biggest baby yet. I breast-fed her while Todd called our family and then we began to talk about and process what had happened.

If I had to relive the same exact scenario, not knowing the outcome was a successful birth; I would still not recognize it as labor. My uterus never felt hard and the pains were localized on the left lower abdomen. They felt so different that with the other two births I had experienced.

The bloody diarrhea was something I have not had before, and it had me scared something was wrong and I was incredibly ill. Therefore, I was not very effective with my relaxation. Had I recognized these as signs of this particular labor, I honestly believe I would have handled the pain more effectively. A part of me was in disbelief that I could have missed the signs of labor. After all, I have given birth twice before and I actually teach natural childbirth education classes. Could I really have been that ignorant? Labor had definitely surprised me and caught me off guard. Whoever said that labor and childbirth was unpredictable was not joking!

The Midwife came into the hospital to examine me and I had no tearing, no hemorrhoids, and no swelling. I was given the choice of going home after the baby was checked out and discharged or if I wanted to stay the night. I decided to stay so the GI doctor could see me for a consult – just to be sure that I was all right. Whether I had a gastroenteritis that put me into labor, or if my body, due to the FM and IBS, just overreacted to the pre-labor prostaglandins and hormones, I will never know. Nevertheless, since I had been sick and was focused on gastrointestinal symptoms, we missed the turning point as to when it changed over to actual labor.

I find it somewhat amusing that since GI problems and pain are such a part of my life, it was possible to actually be in labor but assume it was nothing more that a variation of IBS. Labor is usually one of the most painful and intense experiences of a woman's life and not many miss it's presence and activity in their bodies.

An amazing thing about our story is that I had asked to Todd to make a CD of some of my favorite music for labor. One of my favorite songs on it was "Be Still and Know That I Am God' by Steven Curtis Chapman. It is one of my favorite Bible verses and songs. Right after I delivered, the alarm went off in our bedroom for church and guess which song was playing on the radio? That exact song! We know that was God's way of smiling down on us and our unexpected delivery of our precious little girl, whom we call our "Grand Finale'. I have had a C-section, a vaginal hospital birth, and an unexpected home birth. What else is there left to experience? It has been without a doubt 'quite the ride' and each birth is near and dear to our hearts. We have come a long way on our journey to parenthood and we appreciate and cherish all our childbirth experiences.

Note From Kelly

Whether a pregnant mom or her partner, a childbirth educator, doula, midwife, nurse or doctor, this birth testimony should remind us all that birth is much more than a bodily function. How a woman is treated, how much control she has over the decision-making process, and the words used to describe the problems that arise, all affect who she is as a woman and a mother.

Let us, then, redefine the goal for a healthy mother and baby. Let us include the father into this equation, which equals a healthy new family. May we seek to not only produce a physiological success, but that of an intact body, mind and spirit for all three of them. Perhaps we might be more family-friendly in the delivery room, knowing that the very foundations of family relationships are being formed before us. May we understand that the fabric of society itself is shaped by the love families have for one another, and therefore spend as much resource (if not more) on preserving the heart and spirit of the genesis of the family in the birth room as we do on technology. Perhaps we can invest more time and money into learning how to manage labor without surgical procedures, artificial hormones, electrical devices, and the like.

Stacy's story is an inspiration to us all. She chose to work together with her care providers, rather than against them. She sought to find a peaceable solution to the conflicts that were presented to her, and God honored her gentle and quiet spirit. May we all follow her example.

Epilogue
A Prayer For Families

All the ends of the earth
will remember and turn to the LORD ,
and all the families of the nations
will bow down before him,
for dominion belongs to the LORD
and he rules over the nations.
Psalm 22:27-28 (NIV)

May that be cry of our hearts, Father, that you would have dominion over us. Help us to remember you Lord, and cause each heart to bow down before you. You are the King of pregnancy, God, and we understand that we are fearfully and wonderfully made. You designed us with a fantastic skill that we will never understand, so help us to trust in Your design, to relinquish our control over it, and to dedicate every choice we make to You.

Lord, there is so much to consider during this time, so many schools of thought and so much information out there to soak in. Father, guide and direct Your families, help us to seek after truth and godliness for the sake of our children. Remove any fear or doubt in our minds, for we know that they are not of You. Cause us to be worthy parents of Your children, help us to study and prepare as diligently as we can, because we know that there are things that can snare us. .

Father, equip us with the power of the Holy Spirit so that we can stand firm in the grace of Jesus Christ, as our family grows and develops. Help us to recognize the magnitude of this event, and may we approach it with all seriousness and sobriety. We look forward to seeing your will unfold in our lives, and we desire to be faithful witnesses of Christ, as others watch us while we live our lives out for you. May our testimony be preserved and may we be always sensitive to witnessing to a person who needs You. We all need You, God, and so we are thankful that You have not forsaken us, we are so glad that You keep your promises, and we have faith that You will work out everything that needs to happen in due time.

As we become parents, Lord, may any hidden wound be healed so that we can open up fully to you, giving you full control over our life. Cover our hearts with your healing balm and repair anything that is getting in the way of total surrender to you. We trust in You enough to allow You to restore us, to take control of our life, to take control of this pregnancy and birth, and to take control of our parenting. May we assume the role of parent from the time of conception, nurturing our child with the decisions that we make. May we communicate with them from the beginning and pray for them continually. Let us sing Your praises often so our children will hear them from the womb, and may they recognize the Holy Spirit because He has been within us while they were within us.

We bow down before you Lord, and give you all the glory and honor that you deserve. Be with the families as they remember you during their pregnancy and birth. Allow them to be a witness of your love and grace, the most awesome gift of all. Purify our lives and make us holy, because You are holy. May the words in this book edify, equip, and encourage the reader as they prepare for their child to join them in their arms. When the child looks into their eyes for the first time, may they see You, Holy God. We love You and pray to You in the precious name of Your Son, Jesus Christ. Amen.

Recommended Reading:

40 Weeks:
A Devotional Guide To Pregnancy
By Jennifer Vanderlaan
www.birthingnaturally.net

A Celebration of Pregnancy!
By Doran Richards and Susan Tederick
www.blessingGodsway.com

Childbirth Wisdom
By Judith Goldsmith

Childbirth Without Fear
By Grantly Dick-Read
www.pinterandmartin.com/childbirth.html

Gentle Birth Choices
By Barbara Harper
www.cuttingedgepress.net

Ghosts From The Nursery: Tracing The Roots of Violence
By Robin Karr-Morse & Meredith S. Wiley
www.amazon.com

Pregnancy, Childbirth, & The Newborn
By Penny Simkin
www.cuttingedgepress.net

Supernatural Childbirth
By Jackie Mize

The Lord of Birth
By Jennifer Vanderlaan
www.birthingnaturally.net

The Naturally Healthy Pregnancy: The Essential Guide to Nutritional and Botanical Medicine for the Childbearing Years
By Shonda Parker

The Nurturing Touch at Birth: A Labor Support Handbook
By Paulina (Polly) Perez
www.birthballs.com

When Survivors Give Birth
By Penny Simkin and Phyllis Klaus
www.birthballs.com

Recommended Christian Websites:

www.christianchildbirth.org
www.birthingnaturally.net
www.blessingGodsway.com
www.aboverubies.com
www.gentlebirthchoices.org
www.waterbirth.org
www.gentlemothering.com
www.ChristCenteredChildbirth.com

Early Labor

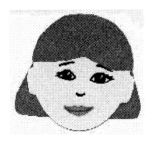

Cervix 0 – 3 cm

Contractions 30 – 45 seconds in length

5 – 30 minutes apart

4 – 12 hours (or more)

- Maintain Normal Activity
- Inform Care Provider
- Nourish yourself and your labor partner
- Make last minute arrangements
- If water breaks, make note of color/odor
- Spend quality time together
- Enjoy a relaxing shower
- Notify loved ones if you so choose
- Avoid going to the hospital too soon
- Time contractions, but do not get preoccupied with them
- Sleep if it is at night

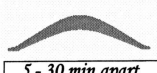 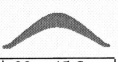

5 - 30 min apart | **30 – 45 Sec**

Contractions are timed from the start of one to the start of the next….

Active Labor

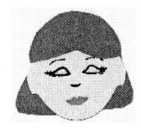

Cervix 4 – 6 cm

Contractions
45– 60 seconds in length

5 – 8 minutes apart

2 – 4 hours (or more)

- Settle into you "nest" where you will be giving birth
- Focus on becoming more tranquil
- Continue to nourish your self to hunger/thirst
- Establish a pattern
- Avoid all unnecessary noise, visitors, and distractions
- Begin abdominal breathing
- Put on worship music
- Maintain a restful state of prayer
- Avoid resisting contractions - surrender

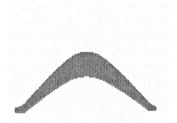

| 5 – 8 Min apart | *45 - 60 Sec* |

Transition

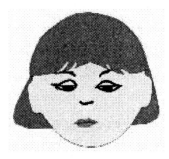

Cervix 7– 10 cm

Contractions
60– 90 seconds in length

1 1/2 – 3 minutes apart

1 – 3 hours

- **Remove all distractions**
- **Strive for total surrender to the power of your body**
- **Reach out to the Lord for your strength**
- **Know that it is almost over**
- **Focus on one contraction at a time**
- **Be mindful of an urge to have a bowel movement and notify your care provider**
- **Pray in the name of the Lord to be confident and allow your body to complete the work it is doing**
- **Remember C.A.L.M.**

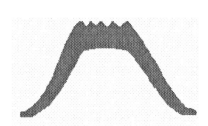
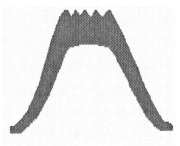

1.5 – 3 minutes between contractions   *60 – 90 Sec.*

Second Stage

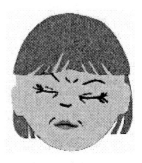

Cervix (gone)

Contractions
60 seconds in length
3– 7 minutes apart

30 min – 3 hours

- Try spontaneous pushing first
- Wait for contraction to build before pushing
- Take in a generous amount of oxygen
- Exhale during push
- If spontaneous efforts are not bringing progress, try a more directed push
- Chin to chest
- Squat during push if possible
- Legs/pelvis open wide
- Perineum relaxed
- Deep vocalization
- Touch head when crowning
- Lift baby to the chest yourself!

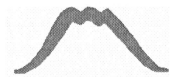

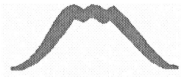

| *3 – 5 minutes apart* | *60 Seconds in length* |

Delivery

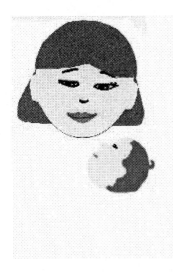

Delivery of Placenta
5 – 45 min

Uterus - Involution

Contractions - Intermittent

Stable in 30 – 60 minutes

- Welcome baby
- Skin-to-skin contact
- Keep baby warm
- Eye-to-eye contact
- No separation for first hour unless ABSOLUTELY necessary
- No pulling on the umbilical cord by attendant
- Wait until the cord stops pulsing before clamping/cutting
- Drink orange juice for quick glucose
- Put warm blankets on mom/baby
- Put baby to the breast
- Get pictures!
- Both parents talk to the baby
- Praise the Lord!

About the Author

Kelly J. Townsend began her childbirth ministry in 1992 as a certified birth doula and childbirth educator in Southern California. After moving to her home state, she went on to serve in the capacity of Doula Coordinator for Ashland Community Hospital in Ashland, OR, as well as acting as a doula/interpretor for the migrant Hispanic women in the community. She served as a Doulas of North America (DONA) trainer and State Representative for Oregon for several years, training and equipping many of the new birth coaches in an era when the title of Doula was almost completely unknown. She studied under Sandra Bardsley, R.N. and Marci Robachaud R.N. through La Clinica Del Valle in Phoenix, OR. Later, Kelly became the Oregon State trainer for Childbirth and Postpartum Professional Association (CAPPA) before deciding that the Lord was leading her into a more specific ministry of Christian Childbirth. Her love of family and concern for other Christian families, and ultimately her love for the Lord fueled her desire to begin a much-needed ministry, devoted to placing Jesus Christ at the center and focus of the birth of a family. Kelly authored Christ Centered Childbirth that has been sold on the internet as an E-Book and desktop copy for five years before formal publishing. The Lord has blessed this book as far away as Croatia, where it is translated into the Croatian language and titled Duhovni pristup radanju, successfully published by a Croatian Christian publisher, Teovizija. She has served as Founder and President of Doulas of Sothern Oregon and is the current Co-Founder and President of Cascade Christian Childbirth Association. Kelly is wife to Dan Townsend and the mother of three naturally born children. She attends Calvary Chapel Tricity in Tempe, AZ and is currently pursuing her Bachelor's degree of Biblical Science at Calvary Chapel Bible College.

Statement of Faith

I and my family believe the following about our best friend, Jesus:

1. Jesus Christ is the son of God, is God, was born of a virgin, was crucified on our behalf as a punishment for the sins of mankind, was resurrected on the third day, ascended into heaven, and is coming back soon to rule and reign for evermore.
2. The only way to eternal salvation is through personal belief that the blood of Jesus is all-sufficient for the penalty of sin and an acceptance of him into your life as Lord and Savior.
3. We believe in salvation by having the faith to believe that it is grace alone that can save us, and that salvation is immediate and eternal upon acceptance of Jesus as a one-time sacrifice for our sins, and not obtained through any works, sacraments, traditions or merits of our own.
4. We believe in the Trinity: That God The Father, God The Son, and God The Holy Spirit are three Persons present in one God.
5. We believe in the eternal and unchanging Word of God, that it is accurate, and infallible. We believe that it is complete, and do not incorporate new age thoughts (Yoga, Unitarianism, Birth Idols, Pagan rituals, Mormonism, Jehovah's Witness, etc.) or Eastern religion into our practice and trust that scripture (as written) is sufficient for any purpose. We are cautious in taking scripture out of context to support an idea, and believe that God can speak to us through scripture individually, yet we do not change the meaning of a passage and declare that it now has a new meaning. Instead, we get to know God's will by seeking to grow in the knowledge of Him and His Son through study of the scriptures.
6. We define "Supernatural Childbirth" as any birth that brings glory to God the Father, regardless of its outcome.
7. We strive to deepen our relationship with Jesus Christ through the childbirth period and to be a witness and testimony to all who God places in our path.
8. We believe that childbirth is a beautiful event that expands far beyond the physical experience, reaching into the very depths of our soul. We also believe that God would have a very special and personal piece of wisdom for us that we would gain from

the experience of our own birth, regardless of how it turned out. We value the presence of the father as an important source of comfort and guidance for the mother, and enjoy seeing the Lord bind their relationship as they become parents. Often times it is the loving eyes of the father that hold her together when things get intense. We understand that when the father cannot be present, the mother can look to Jesus as her comfort and strength.

9. We believe that Satan would desire to use fear and tension to make birth more difficult, in an attempt to turn our birth into a horror story. We also believe that what Satan intended for evil, God can use for good in our lives (Genesis 50:20), so even a very difficult birth can glorify the Lord!

10. We believe that God desires to redeem childbirth so that his children will look first to Him for comfort, support, knowledge, and strength. We also believe that God can give wisdom to our care providers. We strive to see that those attending the birth will seek Godly wisdom and not worldly wisdom so that the best outcome can be achieved. We encourage everyone involved to make educated decisions based on accurate information rather than making rash decisions based on fear.

11. And finally, we pray that each parent and child that the Lord places in our path receives the saving grace of Jesus Christ and that they might come to know Him more intimately through the birth experience!

Come To Know Christ

If you are reading this book and are not Christian, I would like to introduce you to Jesus Christ, the Messiah. Christianity is not only about Heaven, but is about Heaven on Earth. sus willingly was crucified and died on a cross so that you and I could both have an abundant life here on Earth, able to have an intimate relationship with our Creator. We can enjoy an abundant life that, although not free from trial, is full of joy.

Whether you have every material possession, fame, fortune, or power, or have found yourself down and out, there is still a God-shaped hole within you that can only be fulfilled by a close relationship with the Lord. Personal prayer, spiritual ears, discernment of what God might speak to you, and most of all personal peace is overflowing to those who put their trust in the Son of God.

Yes, it was by the sacrifice on the cross that we are able to approach God with boldness and love. That is the first benefit. Even greater is the fact that the blood shed by Jesus Christ is the only thing that can cover our embarrasing record of sin when it comes time to face Father God. We can hide that from our friends and family, but God knows our hearts, the intentions of our heart, and the things that we have done wrong. If we are in a state of sinfulness, God is unable to look upon us in that condition. Since we all have sinned, we all have those stains. There is only one thing that can cover those stains and make them look clean and white, and that is the blood of Jesus.

We can accept the free gift of eternal life, of salvation, and of a life of peace here on Earth, or we can reject it. Christianity isn't about what any of us do, but it is about what He did. He suffered greatly for your sin, so that God would see you as holy. There is nothing greater than a relationship with the Lord, who is living and dynamic and speaks even right now to you, prompting you to accept the gift and open your heart. Why don't you choose today to be cleansed from all guilt and despair, and ask for the peace that passes all understanding? Wouldn't you want that right now? Forget about what others might think. They won't be the ones deciding your eternal future. This is between you and God. Right here, right now.

It is very simple. Jesus' death on the cross was the final sacrifice needed to appease a great God in Heaven. Although many try to deny that fact, the truth is it is going to take your faith to believe it.

You have been saved by grace, that free gift given to you by Jesus, even when you did not deserve it. You accept that gift through faith, not needing to be convinced by scientific evidence. I don't believe anything happens by accident, and I know that by your mere having this book in your hand is a divine appointment for you right now. I suspect that God has been tugging on your heart for some time. Perhaps you once knew God, but turned away for a variety of reasons. Come back to Him. He loves you soooooo much, and wants to have fellowship with you. He wants to hear your prayers once again.

Today is the day for salvation, not tomorrow. Hear the voice of the Lord right now, knocking at your door. It is a still small voice and I believe you can feel it. If you are ready, you can now ask Him to come within you too, so that you might also have a spirit that will come alive. Your life here on earth will be exploding with joy you could have never imagined, even in the middle of trials. Ultimately, you will not perish, but have eternal life; life with the Father. What a glorious day! If you would like to ask the Lord into your heart right now, pray this prayer.

Father God, I can hear you and feel you tugging at my heart. I want that abundant life.. Lord, I don't want hypocrisy or religion, I just want a relationship with you. I know I have sinned, I know I am a sinner. Please forgive me, I don't want to add to the reason you went to the cross, heaping up more sins upon your broken body. Lord, cleanse me now and come within me. Wash me, heal me, and rebuild me so that I might be an effective and useful servant to you. Lord, you know the reasons I have rejected you, and help me to cast those away. I understand that this is about me and you, and about my eternal salvation. I want to live in eternity with you, and I want to be your child. Guide and direct me now as to what I should do next. I love you, Lord. Come into my life. In Jesus' name, Amen!

Welcome to the kingdom!

Suggested Music!

One of the most frequent questions that comes up amongst the ladies on the Christian childbirth yahoo group is what music is good for childbirth. What is important is that the music you listen to during birth should be music that you know and like. You will be more comfortable with familiar surroundings, so if you have been taken out of your home to deliver your baby, familiar music will be a helpful way for you to feel more secure. With that said, I would like to make some suggestions of calming music that is godly and tranquil.

Remember, the music you like in early labor might get chucked out the window during transition. Make sure you bring a variety!

Albums	Artist
Beginnings	Fernando Ortega
(and)	
Camino Largo	(www.fernandoortega.com)
Give You My World	Phil Wickham
	(www.philwickham.com)
In The Quiet Hours –	Phil Keaggy
Instrumental Guitar	
Sleep Sound In Jesus	Michael Card
How Great Is Our God	Passion Worship Band
(For early labor)	

Individual Songs

Deep Enough To Dream	Chris Rice
Lord Move, Or Move Me	FFH
It Is Well With My Soul	Passion Worship Band

I would like to hear from you!

It is always a pleasure to hear from the reader, and I would ask and encourage you to drop me a line to let me know how God has moved in your life.

If you would like me to post your birth story on my website at www.ChristCenteredChildbirth.com, please send it to ChristianChildbirth@yahoo.com via email. All birth stories that will be posted must be submitted electronically.

If you don't have a computer, don't hesitate to send me your comments, questions, or birth story to:

Four Winds Productions
PO Box 3004
Gilbert, AZ 85299

May the Lord truly bless you, and use you as a testimony and witness to those around you, as you bring forth this young life!

For the childbirth professional:

I wholeheartedly encourage you to seek after God's will and plan for your ministry. If you are certain that you have been called to work with young families, then you might consider contacting Cascade Christian Childbirth Association to see how you might get plugged into the ministry. Whether you have been in the field for many years or just starting out, it is good to have a place of sanctuary where God is honored through His Son Jesus Christ.

You will find Cascade at www.ChristianChildbirth.org

May the Lord bless the work of your hands and of your heart, and may you grow deeper in your own walk with Him! Thank you for your heart of ministry!

CASCADE
CHRISTIAN
CHILDBIRTH

www.christianchildbirth.org

Please join me, and every reader of this book, in a moment of worship. Although individually sung at various times, God will knit our voices together into a beautiful tapestry for us to enjoy when we are all together in eternity. If possible, obtain a copy of the music CD "How Great Is Our God" by the Passion Worship Band, which has the following song recorded on it. Listen to that song, and in a state of worship, let's all think of laboring families of old, those giving birth today, and all those in our future who will bring forth God's children. It is an overwhelming and magnificent thing that ties each and every one of us. We truly are one body - may we always give all glory, honor and praise to the Head, Jesus Christ. Praise the Lord!

It Is Well

When peace, like a river, attendeth my way
When sorrows, like sea billows, roll
Whatever my lot, thou hast taught me to say
It is well, it is well with my soul

My sin, o the bliss, of this glorious thought
My sin, not in part, but the whole -
Was nailed to the cross and
I bear it no more - praise the Lord,
Praise the Lord, O my soul

And Lord haste the day
When my faith shall be sight
The clouds be rolled back as a scroll
The trump shall resound and
The Lord shall descend
Even so it is well with my soul

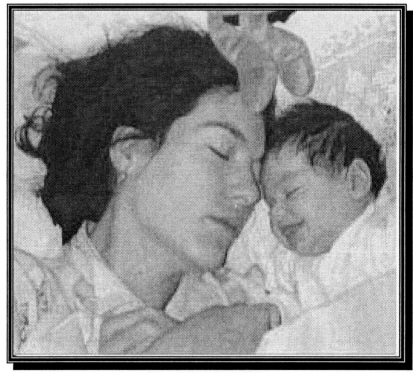

Copyright © 2003

Orders available for discount at:
www.ChristCenteredChildbirth.com

Printed in the United States
60079LVS00005B/22-30

9 780976 950509